Advances in Anatomy, Embryology and Cell Biology
Ergebnisse der Anatomie und Entwicklungsgeschichte
Revues d'anatomie et de morphologie expérimentale

Editors

A. Brodal, Oslo · W. Hild, Galveston · J. van Limborgh, Amsterdam
R. Ortmann, Köln · T. H. Schiebler, Würzburg · G. Töndury, Zürich · E. Wolff, Paris

Advances in Anatomy, Embryology and Cell Biology
Ergebnisse der Anatomie und Entwicklungsgeschichte
Revues d'anatomie et de morphologie expérimentale
Springer–Verlag Berlin Heidelberg GmbH

This journal publishes reviews and critical articles covering the entire field of normal anatomy (cytology, histology, cyto- and histochemistry, electron microscopy, macroscopy, experimental morphology and embryology and comparative anatomy). Papers dealing with anthropology and clinical morphology will also be accepted with the aim of encouraging co-operation between anatomy and related disciplines.

Papers, which may be in English, French or German, are normally commissioned, but original papers and communications may be submitted and will be considered so long as they deal with a subject comprehensively and meet the requirements of the Ergebnisse.

For speed of publication and breadth of distribution, this journal appears in single issues which can be purchased separately; 6 issues constitute one volume.

It is a fundamental condition that manuscripts submitted should not have been published elsewhere, in this or any other country, and the author must undertake not to publish elsewhere at a later date.

25 copies of each paper are supplied free of charge.

Les résultats publient des sommaires et des articles critiques concernant l'ensemble du domaine de l'anatomie normale (cytologie, histologie, cyto et histochimie, microscopie électronique, macroscopie, morphologie expérimentale, embryologie et anatomie comparée. Seront publiés en outre les articles traitant de l'anthropologie et de la morphologie clinique, en vue d'encourager la collaboration entre l'anatomie et les disciplines voisines.

Seront publiés en priorité les articles expressément demandés nous tiendrons toutefois compte des articles qui nous seront envoyés dans la mesure où ils traitent d'un sujet dans son ensemble et correspondent aux standards des «Résultats». Les publications seront faites en langues anglaise, allemande et française.

Dans l'intérêt d'une publication rapide et d'une large diffusion les travaux publiés paraitront dans des cahiers individuels, diffusés séparément: 6 cahiers formen t un volume.

En principe, seuls les manuscrits qui n'ont encore été publiés ni dans le pays d'origine ni à l'étranger peuvent nous être soumis. L'auteur d'engage en outre à ne pas les publier ailleurs ultérieurement.

Les auteurs recevront 25 exemplaires gratuits de leur publication.

Die Ergebnisse dienen der Veröffentlichung zusammenfassender und kritischer Artikel aus dem Gesamtgebiet der normalen Anatomie (Cytologie, Histologie, Cyto- und Histochemie, Elektronenmikroskopie, Makroskopie, experimentelle Morphologie und Embryologie und vergleichende Anatomie). Aufgenommen werden ferner Arbeiten anthropologischen und morphologisch-klinischen Inhaltes, mit dem Ziel, die Zusammenarbeit zwischen Anatomie und Nachbardisziplinen zu fördern.

Zur Veröffentlichung gelangen in erster Linie angeforderte Manuskripte, jedoch werden auch eingesandte Arbeiten und Orginalmitteilungen berücksichtigt, sofern sie ein Gebiet umfassend abhandeln und den Anforderungen der „Ergebnisse" genügen. Die Veröffentlichungen erfolgen in englischer, deutscher und französischer Sprache.

Die Arbeiten erscheinen im Interesse einer raschen Veröffentlichung und einer weiten Verbreitung als einzeln berechnete Hefte; je 6 Hefte bilden einen Band.

Grundsätzlich dürfen nur Manuskripte eingesandt werden, die vorher weder im Inland noch im Ausland veröffentlicht worden sind. Der Autor verpflichtet sich, sie auch nachträglich nicht an anderen Stellen zu publizieren.

Die Mitarbeiter erhalten von ihren Arbeiten zusammen 25 Freiexemplare.

Manuscripts should be addressed to/Envoyer les manuscrits à/Manuskripte sind zu senden an:

Prof. Dr. A. BRODAL, Universitetet i Oslo, Anatomisk Institutt, Karl Johans Gate 47 (Domus Media), Oslo 1/Norwegen

Prof. W. HILD, Department of Anatomy. The University of Texas Medical Branch, Galveston, Texas 77550 (USA)

Prof. Dr. J. van LIMBORGH, Universiteit van Amsterdam, Anatomisch-Embryologisch Laboratorium, Amsterdam-O/Holland, Mauritskade 61

Prof. Dr. R. ORTMANN, Anatomisches Institut der Universität, D-5000 Köln-Lindenthal, Lindenburg

Prof. Dr. T. H. SCHIEBLER, Anatomisches Institut der Universität, Koellikerstraße 6, D-8700 Würzburg

Prof. Dr. G. TÖNDURY, Direktion der Anatomie, Gloriastraße 19, CH-8006 Zürich

Prof. Dr. E. WOLFF, Collège de France, Laboratoire d'Embryologie Expérimentale, 49 bis Avenue de la belle Gabrielle, Nogent-sur-Marne 94/France

Dr. Håkan Aldskogius

Department of Anatomy
Karolinska Institutet
S-104 01 Stockholm 60
Sweden

ISBN 978-3-540-06750-4   ISBN 978-3-642-65867-9 (eBook)
DOI 10.1007/978-3-642-65867-9

Contents

Part I. Indirect Wallerian Degeneration

I. Introduction 7

II. Material and Methods 9

III. Observations 11

   A. Methods 11

   B. Control material (Light and electron microscopy) 11

   C. Experimental material 16

      1. Unoperated side 16

      2. Operated side 16

         a) Light microscopy 17

         b) Electron microscopy 17

           α) Changes in axons and myelin sheats 19

           β) Changes in glial cells and pericytes 21

              Myelin-covered microglial cells 21, Degenerating glial cells 27, Micro-glial cells (outside myelin) 31, Pericytes 31, Mitotic cells 31, Oligodendrocytes 31, Astrocytes 39

           γ) Comparison of results obtained from animals operated on at different ages 39

IV. Discussion 39

   Possible errors in the interpretation of the experimental findings 39

   The experimentally induced degeneration of myelinated nerve fibres 42

   The early reaction of microglial cells 42

   Nature of the degenerating glial cells 45

   The late reaction of microglial cells 47

   The reaction of pericytes 48

   The formation of a glial scar 48

   Possible signs of regenerative activity 49

   Indications concerning the appearance of indirect Wallerian degeneration in adult animals 49

   The dynamic picture of indirect Wallerian degeneration in the kitten — a working hypothesis 50

   The ultrastructural basis of the Nauta picture of indirect Wallerian degeneration 50

   Does the ultrastructural appearance of indirect Wallerian degeneration differ from that of direct Wallerian degeneration? 51

V. Summary 51

Part II. Direct Wallerian Degeneration

I. Introduction 53

II. Material and Methods 53

III. Observations 55
    A. Methods 55
    B. Lesions 55
    C. Changes in the root fibre region on the operated side 56
        a) Light microscopy 56
        b) Electron microscopy 56
            α) Changes in axons and myelin sheats 56
            β) Changes in glial cells 60

IV. Discussion 66
    Limitations inherent in the methods 66
    Comparison between morphological changes during direct and indirect Wallerian
    degeneration 67
    The rate of Wallerian degeneration 69
    Concluding remarks 70

V. Summary 71

Acknowledgement 71

References 71

Subject Index 78

PART I. INDIRECT WALLERIAN DEGENERATION

I. Introduction

After a mechanical lesion of a nerve fibre the part of the fibre distal to the lesion undergoes degenerative changes, so-called Wallerian degeneration. Prominent changes also take place in the fibre parts immediately adjacent to the lesion, the trauma zone (Cajal, 1928a, b). The part of the nerve fibre proximal to the trauma zone can undergo degenerative changes, too (see e.g. Beresford, 1965). These have been shown to be secondary to atrophy and death of the parent cell body of the degenerating fibre (van Gehuchten, 1903) and can thus be regarded as an indirect effect of the lesion of the fibre. Early Marchi studies indicated that although this type of fibre degeneration had a slower time course than Wallerian degeneration distal to the lesion, it had a similar appearance (see e.g. Bregman, 1892, van Gehuchten, 1903). These observations led van Gehuchten (1903) to propose the term *indirect Wallerian degeneration* to describe fibre degeneration between the parent cell body and the trauma zone.

Since the studies of van Gehuchten, indirect Wallerian fibre degeneration has occasionally been reported in the adult nervous system (see e.g. Beresford, 1965; Cole, 1968; Cupédo, 1970; Schlote, 1970; Torvik and Skjörten, 1971; Wong-Riley, 1972). In the immature nervous system, however, it would appear to be a much more common consequence of nerve fibre damage (see Grant, 1970), probably reflecting the fact that immature animals are more liable to react to such damage with nerve cell body death than are adult animals (cf. Brodal, 1939; LaVelle and LaVelle, 1958). In studies in which kittens were used as the experimental material, heavy fibre degeneration was demonstrated with the Nauta method in the intramedullary root fibres of the hypoglossal nerve following peripheral nerve transection (Grant and Aldskogius, 1967), in lumbar spinal ventral root fibres after ventral root or sciatic nerve transection (Grant, 1968), in the cervicothalamic tract after mid-brain lesions (Grant and Westman, 1969) and in the olivo-cerebellar tract after cerebellar lesions (Grant, 1970). Furthermore, it was found that after hypoglossal nerve transection, the degeneration in the intramedullary root fibres of that nerve was preceded by degeneration and ultimately disappearance of cell bodies in the hypoglossal nucleus (Grant and Aldskogius, 1967). Thus it was confirmed that the fibre degeneration occurring between the cell body and the site of lesion is indeed consequent upon death of the parent cell body (cf. van Gehuchten, 1903). The term indirect Wallerian degeneration originally proposed by van Gehuchten, may therefore be considered quite appropriate (Grant and Aldskogius, 1967; Grant, 1970) in contrast to the term retrograde fibre degeneration, which has been used by many authors (see e.g. Beresford, 1965; Cole, 1968). Use of the latter term in this connection is confusing, since it has also been applied to the fibre changes which invariably take place immediately proximal to the lesion (Cajal, 1928a, b). Moreover, the term retrograde fibre degeneration implies that the degeneration proceeds from the site of lesion in the direction of the cell body, but this does not seem to be the case. The available evidence indicates quite to the contrary, that the degeneration proceeds from the cell body in a proximo-distal direction (Bregman, 1892; van Gehuchten, 1903; Glees *et al.* 1951; Cowan *et al.* 1961; Powell and Cowan, 1964; Grant and Aldskogius, 1967). To accord with the terminology proposed above the degenerative changes distal to a nerve fibre lesion should be termed *direct Wallerian* degeneration (see van Gehuchten, 1903).

In kitten material impregnated according to the Nauta technique indirect Wallerian degeneration appears mainly as collections of impregnated granules (Grant and Aldskogius, 1967; Grant, 1968; Grant and Westman, 1969). This contrasts with that of direct Wallerian degeneration, which is characterized predominantly by impregnated fragments of fibre-like structures, an appearance which seems to hold true not only for adult animals but also for kittens (see Grant and Westman, 1969).

The light microscopical appearance of indirect Wallerian fibre degeneration in the kitten has been investigated in great detail. Ultrastructural observations on this type of degeneration are, however, limited to a few brief reports from investigations on adult animals (Takano, 1964; Barron and Doolin, 1968; Schlote, 1970; Torvik and Skjörten, 1971; Wong-Riley, 1972). Further investigation of the fine structural changes associated with this process seems desirable. The knowledge which would accrue would be relevant to our general understanding of the reaction of the central nervous system in various experimental and pathological conditions as well as to the particular question of possible morphological differences between indirect and direct Wallerian degeneration.

The aim of the present study has been to describe the ultrastructural changes in the intramedullary root fibre region of the kitten hypoglossal nerve during indirect Wallerian degeneration. Special attention has been devoted to those aspects of the process which could be directly compared with existing descriptions of direct Wallerian degeneration and also to any changes which might be correlated with previous light microscopical findings on indirect Wallerian degeneration.

The intramedullary root fibres of the kitten hypoglossal nerve were chosen for this investigation for four reasons: 1. Data on the light microscopical appearance of indirect Wallerian degeneration have to a large extent been collected from these fibres. 2. The fibres are considered to be exclusively efferent (for references see Lodge *et al.*, 1973). 3. They are easily identified in slices and sections from the brain stem. 4. Transection of the peripheral hypoglossal nerve is a procedure which can readily be standardized. To find out whether the degree of maturation of the system studied affects the ultrastructural changes produced, kittens of different age groups have been used.

A brief report of some of the changes observed in the present study has been given previously (Aldskogius, 1973).

It will be shown that a characteristic feature of the process of indirect Wallerian degeneration is the occurrence in the region of degenerating fibres of a type of microglial cell completely covered by myelin. The findings indicate that these cells reach their position inside myelin by a process of active migration,

Table 1. Summary of time data for animals subjected to hypoglossal nerve transection

	Age at op. (days)	Survival time (days)	No. of animals
Group I	2– 7	1–60	35
Group II	10–17	1–60	13
Group III	21–28	4–30	10

that they participate in the phagocytosis of degenerating axoplasm and that they in turn degenerate and are eliminated. From a survey of the relevant litterature it appears that myelin-covered microglial cells of the type described in the present study have not been unequivocally linked before with direct Wallerian degeneration. Whether this type of cell is a characteristic feature of indirect Wallerian degeneration in the kitten cannot be decided at present, due to insufficient knowledge about the early glial reaction during direct Wallerian degeneration in the cat.

II. Material and Methods

73 kittens were used for the present study. 58 of these animals were subjected to operation and served as experimental material. 15 non-operated animals served as control material. While a minority of the kittens had an exactly known age at operation, the ages of the remainder had to be calculated on the basis of information from suppliers. Based on age at operation the operated animals were arbitrarily separated into three groups (Table 1). The ages of the non-operated animals ranged from 1 to 60 days.

The animals were anaesthetized with Mebumal® (30 mg/kg) i.p. sometimes supplemented with 0.5–1.0 ml Xylocain-Exadrin® (Astra, Södertälje, Sweden) administered locally. With sterile precautions, the right hypoglossal nerve was exposed where it passes below the posterior belly of the digastric muscle and was severed with a pair of scissors, avoiding any traction of the nerve. About 5 mm of the nerve were resected. After the animals has been killed, the operation area was inspected macroscopically. In all cases the operated nerve seemed to be completely severed.

All the animals were given penicillin intramuscularly in the gluteal region immediately after the operation. The animals seemed to be in good condition throughout the whole of the postoperative period.

All the animals were killed by perfusion under Mebumal® anaesthesia. The perfusion procedure was as follows: The chest was opened and a cannula inserted into the ascending aorta via the left chamber of the heart. Thereafter the right atrium was opened and the descending aorta clamped just above the diaphragm. A rinsing solution was perfused at pressure of 100–120 mm Hg for about 30 secs. After the rinse a fixative solution with a temperature of 38°C was perfused for 3–4 min at a pressure of 100–120 mm Hg. This solution was followed by cold (7°C) fixative solution perfused for 12–15 min, either at a constant pressure of 70–100 mm Hg (36 operated, 10 non-operated animals) or at a discontinuous pressure (cf. Berthold, 1968; Hildebrand, 1971a) varying between 90 and 20 mm Hg (22 operated, 5 non-operated animals). Both the rinsing and fixative solutions had a pH of 7.35–7.45.

Various rinsing and fixative solutions were used (Table 2).

After perfusion the lower brain stem and upper spinal cord were carefully dissected out. This material was put in a cold (7°C) fixative solution of the same composition as had been used for the perfusion fixation but without Dextran, stored in this solution in the refrigerator for a few hours or days and then cut transversely into slices approximately 1 mm thick. From these slices, blocks containing the intramedullary root fibre region of the hypoglossal nerve were cut out bilaterally under a dissection microscope. Neither the region

Table 2. Rinsing solutions and fixative solutions used for perfusion of the experimental (op.) and the control (non-op.) material used in the study

Rinsing solution	Tonicity (mOsm)	Fixative solution	Tonicity (mOsm)	No. of aimals op.	non-op.
Sörensen phosphate buffer	400–450	2 % glutaraldehyde 1 % formaldehyde 100 mOsm cacodylate buffer	700–750	8	2
Millonig buffer+ 2.7 % Dextran T 40	300	2 % glutaraldehyde 1 % formaldehyde 300 mOsm Millonig buffer+2.7 % Dextran T 40	850–890	20	6
Millonig buffer + 2.7 % Dextran T 40	300	5 % glutaraldehyde 300 mOsm Millonig buffer+2.7 % Dextran T 40	800–850	30	7

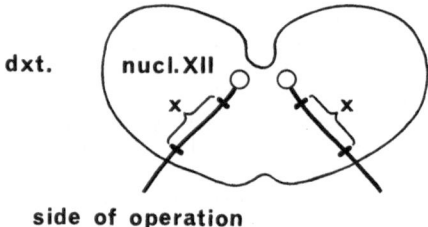

Fig. 1. Schematic drawing of a transverse section through the medulla oblongata of the kitten. × shows the region of the intramedullary root fibres of the hypoglossal nerve which was prepared for light and electron microscopy

close to the nucleus nor the region close to the ventral surface of the medulla was included (cf. Fig. 1). During the latter procedure the slices were kept at room temperature in the rinsing solution previously used during perfusion (without Dextran). The blocks taken from the root fibre regions were divided into smaller blocks representing various proximo-distal parts of the intramedullary portion of the nerve. In some cases blocks were prepared only from slices containing the rostral half of the root fibres. In these instances the caudal half of the root fibre region was used for another study (Aldskogius, to be published).

The small blocks were rinsed either in Sörensen or Millonig buffer (1961), depending upon which rinsing solution had been used at perfusion (cf. Table 2). They were then post-fixed for 2 hrs in 1 % osmium tetroxide in Sörensen or Millonig buffer, dehydrated in a graded series of ethanol and embedded in Epon 812. The blocks were oriented so that both transversely and longitudinally cut sections of the intramedullary root fibres were obtained. 1 μm thick sections were cut from every single small block both from the experimental and from the control animals. The sections were stained with toluidine blue and examined with the light microscope. This was done to evaluate the appearance of the normal and the degenerating structures and to select representative areas from the blocks for further processing for electron microscopy. Sections from the unoperated side of the experimental material were used mainly for making a light microscopical comparison with the operated side. Blocks from the unoperated sides of 12 animals, 5–24 days old at operation and with survival times varying between 6 and 60 days were further processed for electron microscopy. Short series (20–30 sections) of silver-grey sections were made on an LKB Ultrotome from the small blocks of the cases prepared for electron microscopy. In addition, longer series (300–400 sections) were made from small blocks of many cases. The sections were mounted on one-hole formvar-coated copper grids, stained with uranyl acetate and lead citrate (Reynolds, 1963) or with lead citrate alone and examined in a Philips 300 EM electron microscope at an accelerating voltage of 80 kV.

III. Observations

A. Methods (cf. Table 2)

The most uniform preservation was obtained after perfusion with 5% glutaraldehyde solution. The other two fixative solutions gave satisfactory preservation of all tissue constituents with the exception of myelin sheaths. When the vehicle for the fixative was a 300 mOsm Millonig buffer solution the latter often showed some splitting of their lamellae and use of a 100 mOsm cacodylate buffer solution often caused still more extensive splitting. No differences were apparent between material which had been perfused with cold fixative solution at a constant pressure and material which had been perfused at a discontinuous pressure.

B. Control Material

Light and Electron Microscopy

Fig. 2a—e give a general idea of the normal postnatal development of the intramedullary root fibres of the hypoglossal nerve. During the first few days after birth unmyelinated fibres and small myelinated fibres (Fig. 2a) can be seen. One week after birth myelinated fibres constitute the great majority of the intramedullary root fibres (Fig. 2b). At two weeks unmyelinated fibres are extremely rare (Fig. 2c). Growth was found to continue throughout the whole period studied (Fig. 2a—e). The axons displayed the same ultrastructural morphology as has been described previously (see e.g. Peters et al., 1970). The myelin sheaths showed a lamellar configuration with a repeating period of 90–110 Å when measured on fibres 2–4 μm thick.

Three types of glial cells were observed.

The most frequently seen glial cell type was a dark type (Fig. 3), which was considered to correspond to the oligodendrocyte described by previous authors (see e.g. Mugnaini and Walberg, 1964; Kruger and Maxwell, 1966; Wendell-Smith et al., 1966; Bunge, 1968; Mori and Leblond, 1970; Lyser, 1972). It was characterized by a slightly irregular outline with many short processes (Fig. 3). The nucleus was round or oval and displayed a high electron density with slight or moderate condensation of chromatin beneath the nuclear membrane (Fig. 3). The nucleolus was often prominent (Fig. 3). In the electron-dense cytoplasm the following features were noted: a rather well-developed rough endoplasmic reticulum, numerous free ribosomes, round mitochondria with poorly defined cristae and a Golgi apparatus with rather wide cisterns (Fig. 3). Microtubules were often seen. In some instances the cell membrane was continuous with the outer myelin lamella of at least one adjacent nerve fibre.

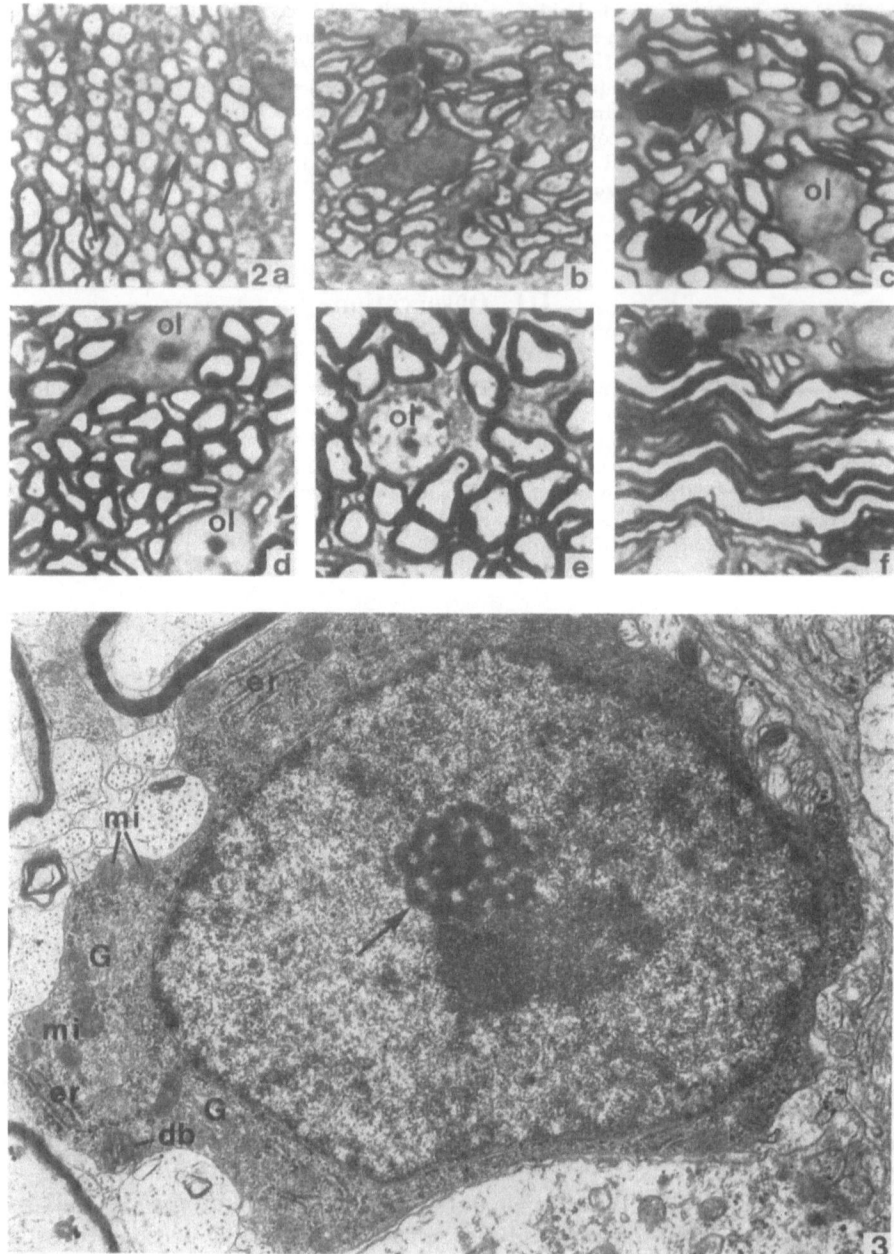

Fig. 2a—f. Control material from kittens of various ages. Light micrographs from 1 μm thick
toluidine-blue stained, transverse (a–e) and longitudinal (f) sections of the intramedullary root
fibre region of the hypoglossal nerve. × 1650. a 3 days, b 7 days, c 14 days, d 23 days,
e 60 days, f 23 days. Fig. 2a—e show the gradual increase in the mean size of the nerve fibres
and myelin sheaths. In Fig. 2a the myelinated nerve fibres are intermingled with fibres which
seem to be unmyelinated (arrows). In Fig. 2b, the great majority of the nerve fibres are
myelinated and in Fig. 2c, no unmyelinated fibres cen be seen. Arrowheads in Fig. 2a, b and f
point at dark, irregularly outlined formations, which in the electron microscope turned out
to be myelin bodies. Note glial cells (ol), probably oligodendrocytes

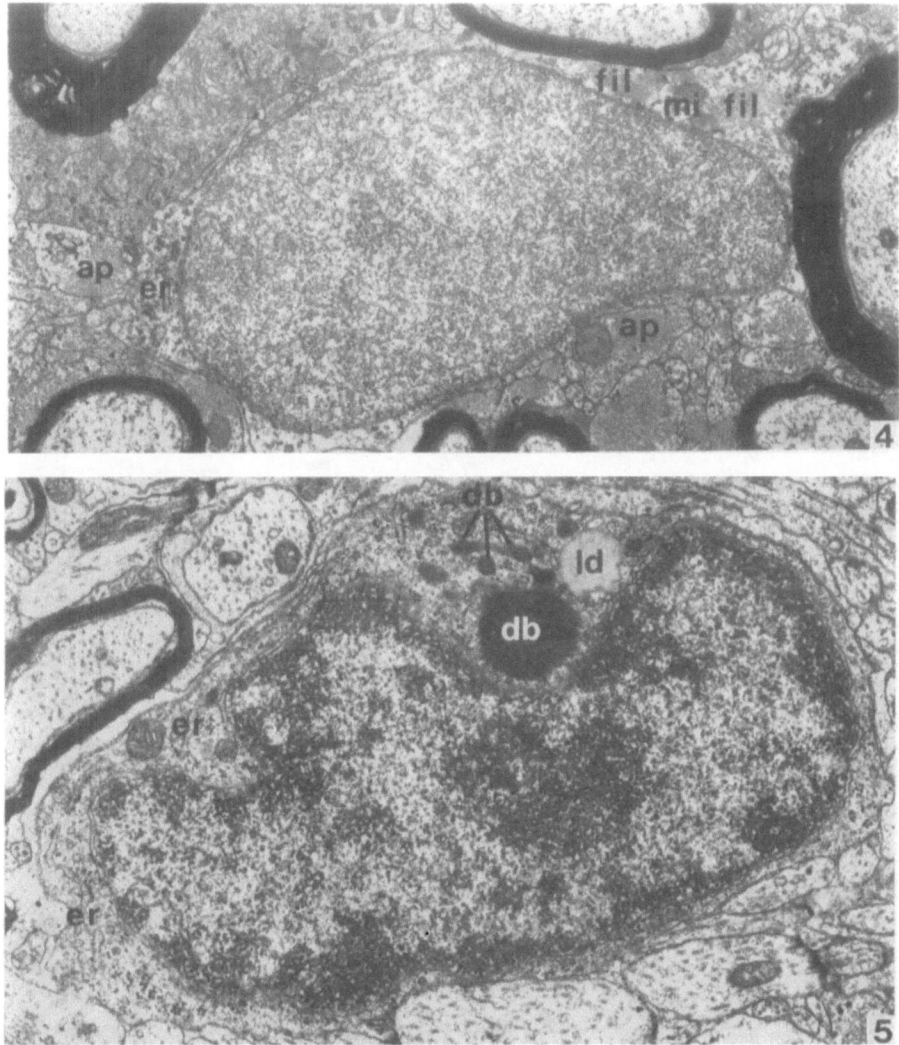

Fig. 4. Control material. 14 days. Astrocyte with an oval, pale nucleus and a pale cytoplasm in which scattered ribosomes, a few short membranes of rough-surfaced endoplasmic reticulum (*er*), two mitochondria (*mi*) and a few short bundles of filaments (*fil*) are seen. Close to the cell are several astocytic processes (*ap*) to a large extent filled with filaments. × 12 000

Fig. 5. Control material. 23 days. Microglial cell with elongated somewhat indented nucleus in which marked clumping of chromatin is seen. The cytoplasm is less electron-dense than the nucleus. Small groups of ribosomes are scattered in the cytoplasm, which in addition contains a few single rows of rough-surfaced endoplasmic reticulum (*er*), several dense bodies (*db*) and one lipid droplet (*ld*). × 17 750

Fig. 3. Control material. 5 days. Oligodendrocyte with an electron-dense nucleus showing moderate clumping of chromatin and a conspicuous nucleolus (arrow). In the electron-dense cytoplasm numerous free ribosomes cen be seen. The rough-surfaced endoplasmic reticulum (*er*) is rather well developed, the mitochondria are characteristically plump (*mi*) and the Golgi apparatus (*G*), which is not very prominent, consists of rather wide cisterns. Note heterogeneous dense body (*db*). × 15 000

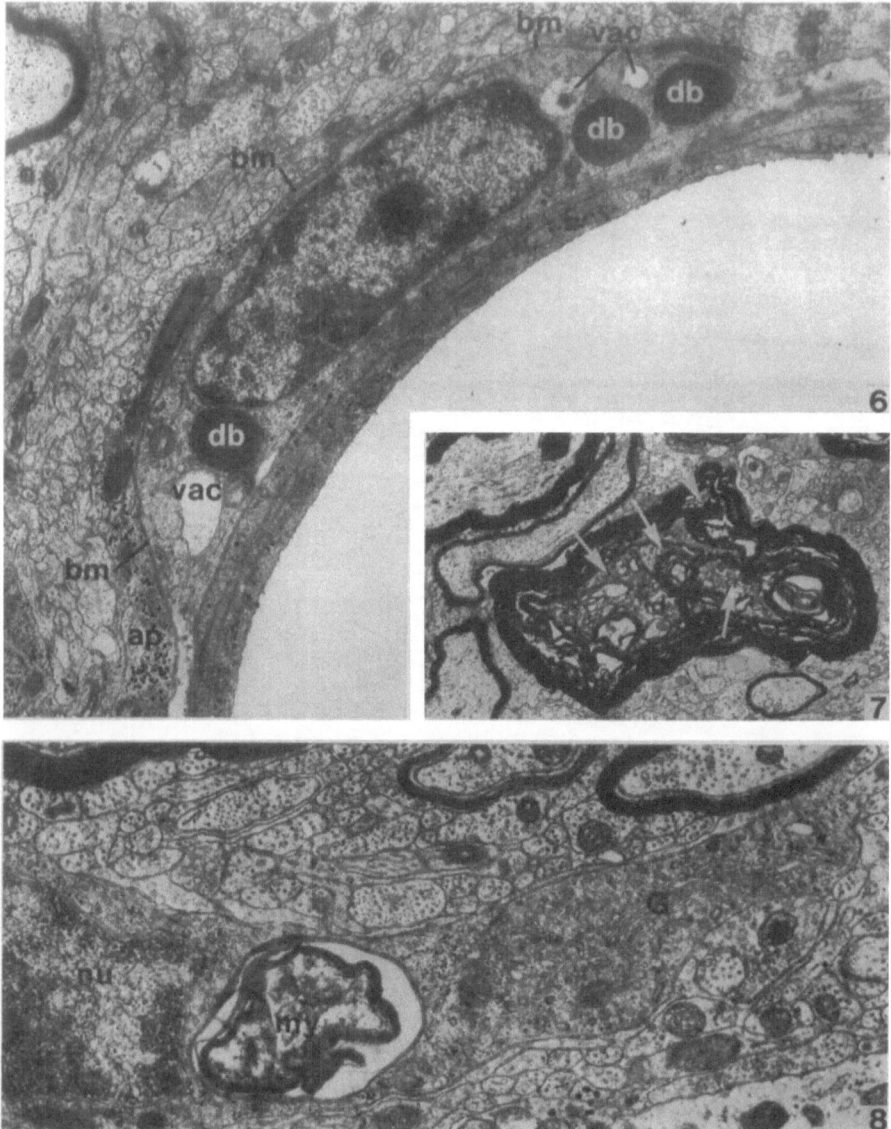

Fig. 6. Control material. 23 days. Pericyte, completely enveloped by basement membrane (*bm*). The nucleus is electron-dense and shows clumps of chromatin. In the cytoplasm there are three dense bodies (*db*) and three vacuoles (*vac*). An astrocytic process (*ap*) filled with glycogen granules can be seen adjacent to the basement membrane. × 10650

Fig. 7. Control material. 14 days. Myelin body. A few layers of myelin are irregularly wrinkled and folded. Electron-dense granular and partially vacuolated cytoplasmic-like material can be seen in the centre and also at the periphery (arrows). × 10650

Fig. 8. Control material. 23 days. Microglial cell with elongated outline. The visible part of the nucleus (*nu*) shows clumps of chromatin. The cytoplasm, which has an electron density intermediate between the nucleus and the neuropil adjacent to the cell, contains a well developed Golgi apparatus (*G*) consisting of a few flattened cisterns and several vesicles. A myelin-like structure (*my*) has been engulfed by the cell. × 18000

Far less common than this dark type of glial cell was a light type (Fig. 4). This was similar to the astrocyte of previous descriptions (see e.g. Mugnaini and Walberg, 1964; Maxwell and Kruger, 1965; Wendell-Smith *et al.*, 1966; Mori and Leblond, 1969b; Lyser, 1972). The identification of these cells and their processes was above all based on the occurrence of bundles of filaments (Fig. 4). In addition, this cell type was characterized by a lower cytoplasmic and nuclear electron density than the oligodendrocyte (Fig. 4). The usually oval nucleus displayed a more or less evenly dispersed chromatin (Fig. 4) and an inconspicuous nucleolus. The cytoplasm contained relatively few organelles (Fig.4).

The least common glial cell type had the following characteristics: the nucleus and the cell body had an elongated, often irregular outline (Fig. 8). The electron density of the nucleus was high and there were prominent, peripherally located chromatin condensations (Figs. 5 and 8). The nucleolus was often inconspicuous. The often scanty cytoplasm had a much lower density than the nucleus (Figs. 5 and 8). The cytoplasm contained only few membranes of rough-surfaced endoplasmic reticulum, scattered small groups of ribosomes (Fig. 5), a Golgi apparatus with narrow cisterns (Fig. 8), lipid droplets and dense bodies (Fig. 5). The mitochondria were elongated with distinct cristae. The similarities between these cells and cells designated as microglial cells by previous authors (see e.g. Blakemore, 1969; Mori and Leblond, 1969a; Vaughn and Peters, 1971; Mugnaini, 1972; Vaughn and Skoff, 1972; Phillips, 1973) were striking. Therefore, the third glial cell type described here will be termed microglial cell regardless of its embryogenetic origin.

Pericytes displayed an elongated dark nucleus with chromatin aggregations beneath the nuclear membrane (Fig. 6). The relatively scanty, medium-dark cytoplasm contained a few stacks of roughsurfaced endoplasmic reticulum, free ribosomes, vesicles and sometimes a few vacuoles and dense bodies (Fig. 6).

Occasional mitotic cells were seen.

Signs of myelin sheath and glial cell degeneration were found in the control material.

In the toluidine-blue light microscope sections occasional dark, irregularly outlined structures were observed (Fig. 2b, c and f). In the electron microscope these structures were found to represent irregularly outlined bodies consisting of myelin layers wrinkled and folded upon each other (Fig. 7). These structures will be referred to as myelin bodies (cf. Hildebrand, 1971a, b). Cytoplasmic-like material was seen in their centre (Fig. 7) and sometimes also between some of their different myelin layers (Fig. 7, arrows). The nature of this material could not be established.

Occasionally, myelin-like bodies were found within microglial cells, apparently having been engulfed (Fig. 8). Clearly degenerating axons, i.e. electron-dense axons (see e.g. Guillery, 1970) filamentous axons (cf. Mugnaini and Walberg, 1967) or electron-lucent axons (cf. O'Neal and Westrum, 1973) were not found.

Aberrant myelin i.e. double layers of myelin forming loops were occasionally found to surround normal-looking oligodendrocytes (Fig. 9).

During the first 23 days one or a few structures interpreted as degenerating glial cells were found in most control animals. They all seemed to be in an advanced stage of degeneration. A pyknotic nucleus and disintegrated cytoplasm character-

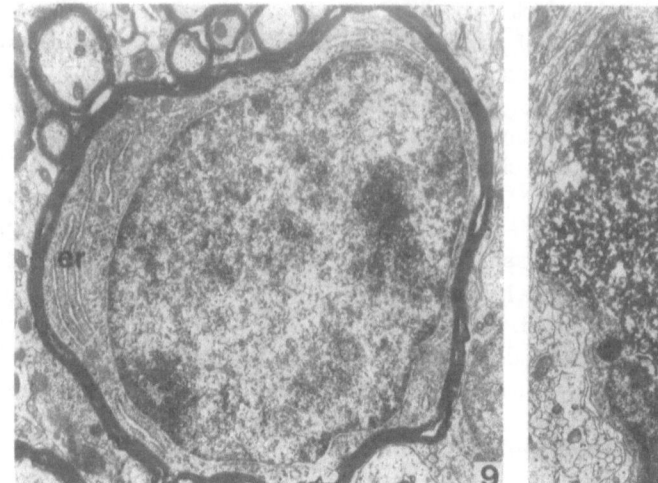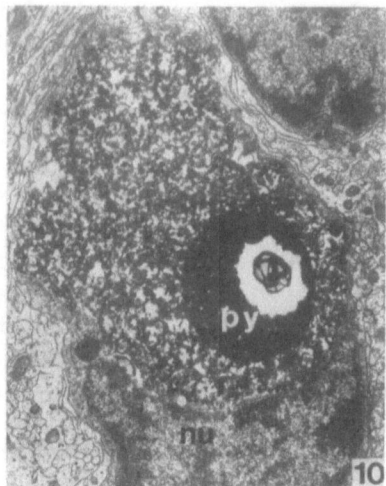

Fig. 9. Control material. 39 days. An oligodendrocyte surrounded by aberrant myelin. Note characteristic endoplasmic reticulum (*er*). × 9000

Fig. 10. Control material. 23 days. Structure interpreted as degenerating glial cell has been engulfed by a microglial cell, the nucleus of which is partially visible (*nu*). The large, dense, vacuolated body (*py*) may be the remains of the nucleus of the degenerating cell and the disintegrated area the remains of its cytoplasm. × 7100

ized all these cells (Fig. 10), the exact identity of which could not be established. A few of them were phagocytosed by microglial cells (Fig. 10).

C. Experimental Material

1. Unoperated Side

No differences in the number and appearance of myelin bodies and degenerating glial cells were detected between the unoperated side and the control material.

2. Operated Side

In the following description the time data for the appearance of the changes described refer to the youngest group of kittens (cf. Table 1). In this group the number of degenerating fibres seemed to be largest. With regard to the appearance of the degenerative changes, however, the three groups of animals will not be dealt with separately, since the observations were essentially similar in all three groups.

a) Light Microscopy

Darkly stained axons (Fig. 11a, e and f) were observed from 3 to 35 days postoperatively. Irregularly outlined dark formations (Fig. 11e and f) reminiscent of the myelin bodies seen in the control material were more numerous than usual from 7 to 35 days. These formations seemed to be most frequent about 2 to 3 weeks postoperatively. Aberrant myelin (Fig. 11 c and d) was regularly observed from 8 to 35 days.

Glial cells surrounded by myelin were observed from 3 to 35 days. Many of these cells had a heterochromatic nucleus and were elongated in sections cut longitudinally with respect to the root fibres (Fig. 11 b). Other cells had an euchromatic nucleus and a rounded appearance (Fig. 11 c). By examination of serial 1 μm thick sections the last-mentioned cell type was found to be only partially covered by myelin (Fig. 11 c and d).

Structures interpreted as degenerating glial cells were observed in increased numbers from 8 to 60 days. These structures displayed a large pyknotic body surrounded by disintegrated and/or vacuolated material and were usually bordered by myelin (Fig. 11 f, g, h and i).

Glial cells with vacuoles and inclusions were observed regularly from 9 to 35 days, particularly about 2 to 3 weeks postoperatively (Fig. 11 i).

By 60 days there was an apparent reduction in the number of nerve fibres in the intramedullary portion of the hypoglossal nerve (cf. Figs. 2 e and 11 i).

b) Electron Microscopy

Diagram 1 summarizes the first appearance and duration of some of the most conspicuous changes on the operated side of the experimental material.

Diagram 1. First appearance and duration of some of the most conspicuous ultrastructural changes which were observed in myelinated nerve fibres and glial cells following ipsilateral hypoglossal nerve transection in kittens aged 2–7 days at operation. Areas with hatched lines indicate the time periods when the different changes were most frequently observed

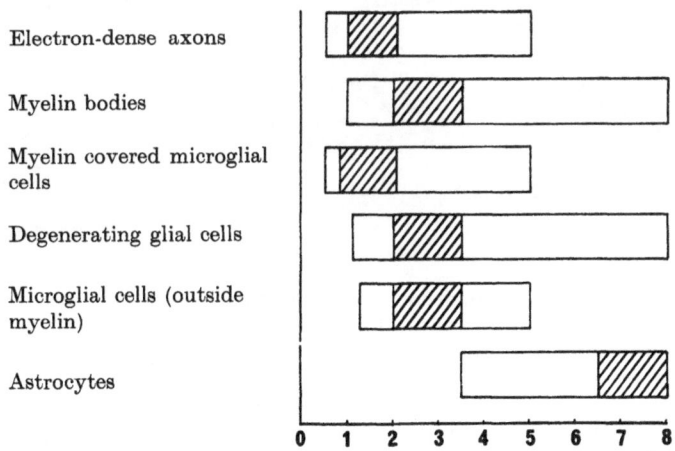

Postoperative survival time
(weeks)

18 H. Aldskogius

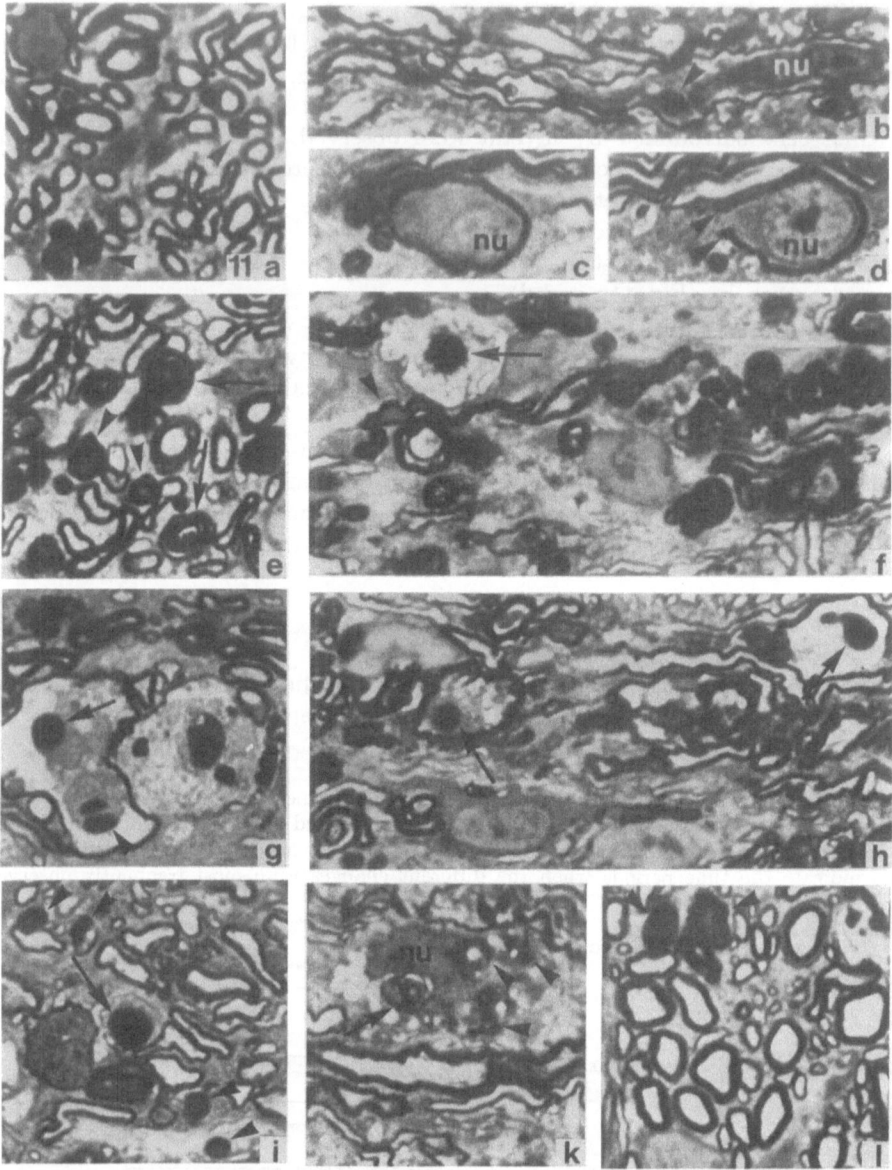

Fig. 11 a—l. Experimental material, operated side. Light micrographs of 1 µm thick, toluidine-blue stained sections. × 1650. a 4 days at operation, 3 days survival. Transverse section. Three darkly stained axons are seen (arrowheads). b The same case as in Fig. 11 a. Longitudinal section. An elongated glial cell with heterochromatic nucleus (*nu*) is covered by myelin. A dark inclusion (arrowhead) is seen in the cytoplasm of the cell. c, d 5 days at operation, 8 days survival. Longitudinal section. Two sections 1 µm apart. A loop of double-layered myelin (aberrant myelin) is partially surrounding a glial cell with an euchromatic nucleus (*nu*), probably an oligodendrocyte. The outer and inner myelin layers are continuous with each other (arrowheads). e 6 days at operation, 9 days survival. Transverse section. Two darkly stained axons are seen (arrowheads). In addition several rounded or irregular formations can be seen (arrows), some of them having alternating dark and light zones. f The same case as in Fig. 11 e. Longitudinal section. A large number of dark, rounded or irregularly outlined formations are α) **Changes in Axons and Myelin Sheaths.** From 3 to 7 days axons were seen in which filaments and tubules were unusually tightly packed and the mitochondria seemed to be enlarged (Fig. 13).

Electron-dense axons were the ultrastructural counterparts of the dark axons seen with the light microscope. Whilst rarely seen at 3 and 4 days, electron-dense axons were observed more regularly from the 5th day onwards and seemed to be most frequent between 7 and 15 days. They were never dominant among degenerating structures as a whole. The electron density of these axons was due to their homogeneously dark axoplasm, in which neither filaments nor tubules could be observed (Figs. 14 and 15). The mitochondria often seemed swollen and their cristae disintegrated (Figs. 14 and 15). Vesicular structures, vacuoles dense profiles (Fig. 4) and membranous formations (Fig. 15) were occasionally observed within the electron-dense axons. The myelin surrounding the electron-dense axons appeared normal (Fig. 14). In some instances loosening of the myelin lamellae was seen (Fig. 15).

Many electron-dense axons gave the impression of having undergone shrinkage (Fig. 12). In several axons it was obvious that the aoxplasm was shrunken and/or disintegrated. Shrinkage of the axoplasm was usually accompanied by wrinkling and ultimately collapse of the surrounding myelin to form myelin bodies (Figs. 12 and 16). Occasionally, however, extensive shrinkage and even complete absence of axoplasm was noted inside a normal-looking myelin sheath (Fig. 13).

In some animals dilated fibres were seen with a core of tightly packed filaments, which were centrally located (Fig. 18). Around this core, tubular profiles, mitochondria of very variable appearance, dense bodies, vesicles and lamellated structures were found (Fig. 18). In a few of these fibres a microglial cell was seen lying between the axoplasm and the myelin sheath.

seen in the picture, particularly to the right. One darkly stained axon can be seen (arrowhead). At upper left, a large pyknotic structure (arrow) surrounded by a faintly stained area with an irregular outline, which in turn seems to be surrounded by an "empty" area. g 5 days at operation, 15 days survival. Transverse section. To the left, a greatly distended myelin sheath, in which a single, round pyknotic body (arrow) and a group of two large, elongated pyknotic bodies (arrowhead) occur. The single body is surrounded by a partially vacuolated structure. The group of two bodies is surrounded by a round homogeneous structure. To the right, a large, vacuolated structure containing one large, dark body and two smaller ones and at some places bordered by myelin. h The same case as in Fig. 11g. Longitudinal section. A few fragments of fibres are visible. In addition there are two pyknotic bodies (arrows). The one on the left is surrounded by a vacuolated area. The one on the right is surrounded by an empty-looking area. Note myelin in the periphery of both areas. i 7 days at operation, 25 days survival. Transverse section. A few fragments of fibres are visible (arrowheads). In the middle of the picture a large, dark body (arrow) with a rather thin light zone around it. To the left of that body a distended myelin sheath containing dark material in which a few small light and dark profiles can be seen. k The same case as in Fig. 11i. Longitudinal section. Glial cell (nucleus = nu) with numerous lipid inclusions, one large, dark inclusion (arrow) and several small dense bodies (arrowheads). l 5 days at operation, 60 days survival. Transverse section. Upper left, two fragments of myelinated fibres (arrowheads). The picture shows nearly all the myelinated nerve fibres which existed in one "fascicle" of the intramedullary root fibres of the hypoglossal nerve at this postoperative stage. By comparison with Fig. 2e, which shows only a small part of such a fascicle at a similar age of the animal, it is apparent that a reduction in the number of fibres has occurred

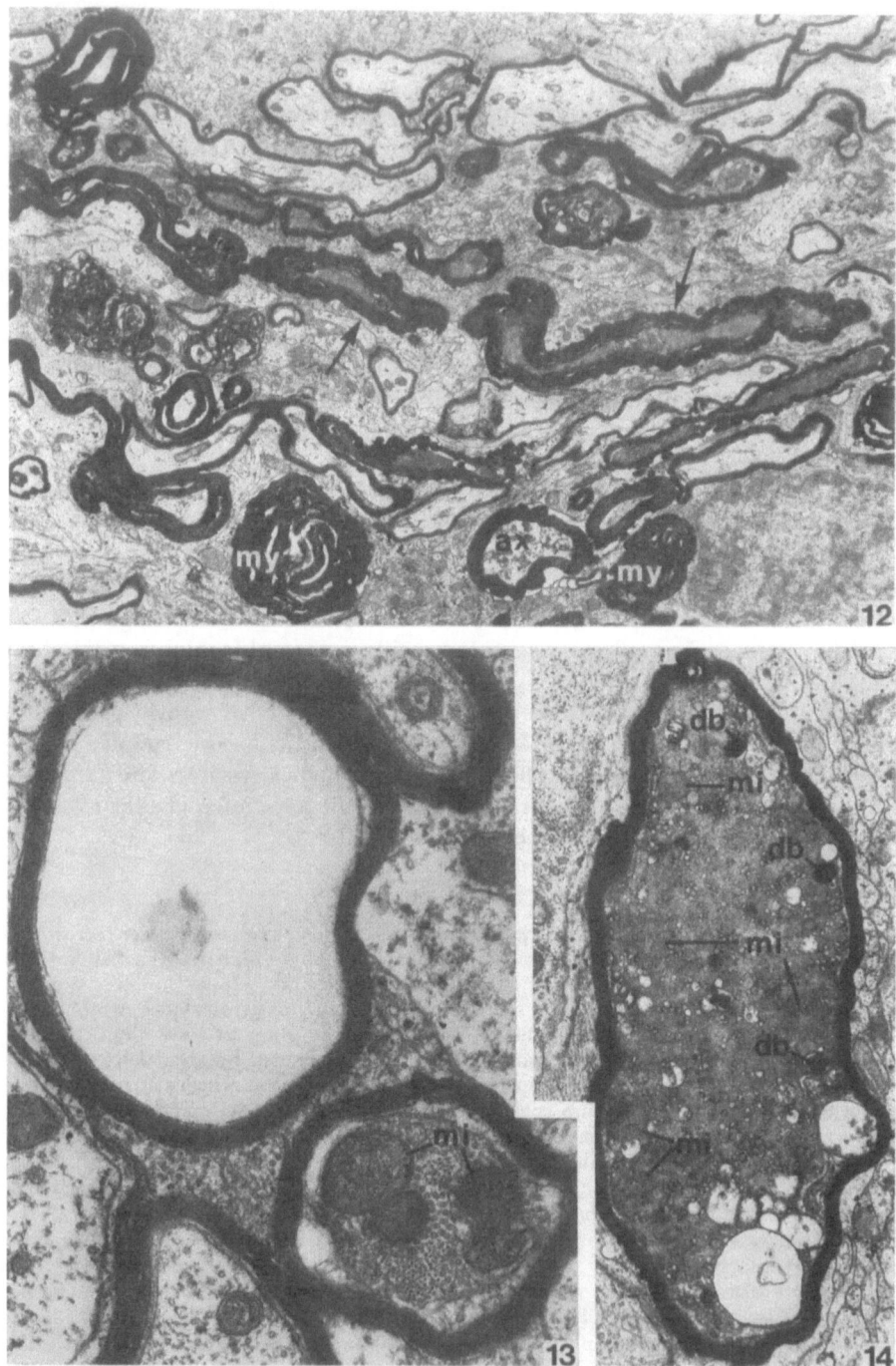

Fig. 12. 7 days at operation, 15 days survival. Longitudinal section. Several myelinated nerve fibres with electron-dense axoplasm. Moderate shrinkage of axoplasm and loosening of the surrounding myelin lamellae can be seen in some fibres (arrows). In one fibre (ax) the axoplasm is dissoluted. The myelin surrounding it is somewhat wrinkled. Two myelin bodies (my) consisting of several layers of collapsed myelin can be seen. × 5600

Two types of myelin sheath degeneration were observed; myelin bodies and aberrant myelin.

In the electron microscope the dark, irregularly outlined structures seen in the light microscope were found to be myelin bodies (see above). They were seen throughout the whole of the period studied. They were more numerous from 7 to 35 days than in the control material or the unoperated side of the experimental material. They seemed to be most frequent from 2 to 3 weeks. Thereafter their number declined. The myelin bodies were of various sizes and forms, but usually they were rounded or elongated. The myelin period was usually normal (Fig. 16 inset). Granular or disintegrated cytoplasmic-like material was usually found between the myelin layers in the central region of the bodies and often also between peripheral layers (Fig. 16). The nature of the centrally located cytoplasmic-like material could not be established. Some pictures suggested that the peripherally located material consisted of oligodendroglial cell cytoplasm (Fig. 16).

Aberrant myelin was sometimes seen surrounding apparently normal oligodendroglial cells (Fig. 17). An opening was invariably found in this myelin covering at which location the inner and outer myelin layers were seen to be continuous with each other (cf. Fig. 11 c and d).

β) Changes in Glial Cells and Pericytes (cf. Diagram 1).

Myelin-covered Microglial Cells

From 3 to 35 days postoperatively microglial cells were observed to be enclosed by myelin sheaths. At 5 to 15 days such cells were common, particularly during the first few days of this period.

In single sections, transversely or longitudinally cut in relation to the root fibres, the cells were with few exceptions completely covered by myelin. Serial sections through some of these cells showed them to be entirely ensheathed by myelin. Occasionally two microglial cells were observed inside the same myelin sheath (Fig. 21). In most instances the covering myelin appeared normal (Figs. 19, 20, 22a and b). Occasionally it was thin, irregular and only partially covering the cell (Fig. 23). In a few cases the innermost lamellae were detached from the rest of the surrounding myelin (Fig. 34).

In longitudinal sections of the intramedullary root fibres the glial cells were usually elongated (Figs. 20 and 22), whereas in transverse sections they were usually rounded (Fig. 19). The nucleus was electron-dense, irregular and showed peripheral chromatin aggregations (Figs. 19, 20, 21, 22a and 23). The nucleolus was not very prominent. The cytoplasm was abundant, with numerous processes. These often seemed to be tightly packed and sometimes invaginated the cytoplasm of the parent cell (Figs. 19 and 22a) or of another glial cell located within the same myelin sheath (Fig. 21). In some instances the processes radiated freely

Fig. 13. 2 days at operation, 7 days survival. Transverse section. Upper left, apparently normal myelin surrounding an "empty" space. Lower right, myelinated axon with two enlarged mitochondria (mi) without clearly visible cristae and with tightly packed filaments and tubules. × 36000

Fig. 14. 4 days at operation, 3 days survival. Longitudinal section. Electron-dense axon containing several vacuoles of various sizes and five just visible mitochondria (mi). In addition several small dense profiles can be seen (db). × 12000

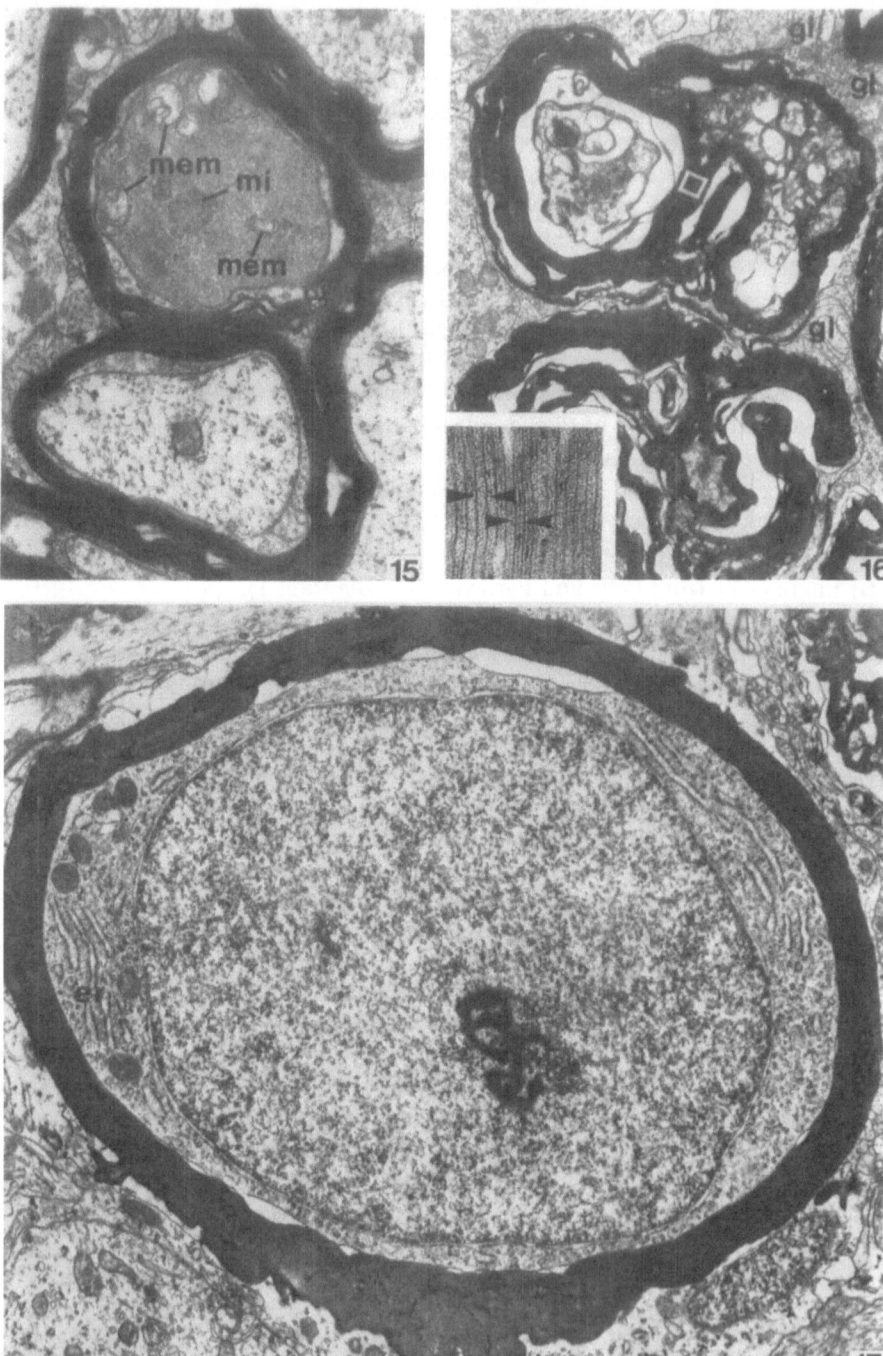

Fig. 15. 15 days at operation, 9 days survival. Transverse section. Above, electron-dense axon containing one mitochondrion (*mi*) in which cristae are not clearly visible. In addition several membranous profiles (*mem*) are seen. Compared to the surrounding apparently normal myelinated axons, there seems to be some loosening of the myelin lamellae around the electron-dense axon. × 18 000

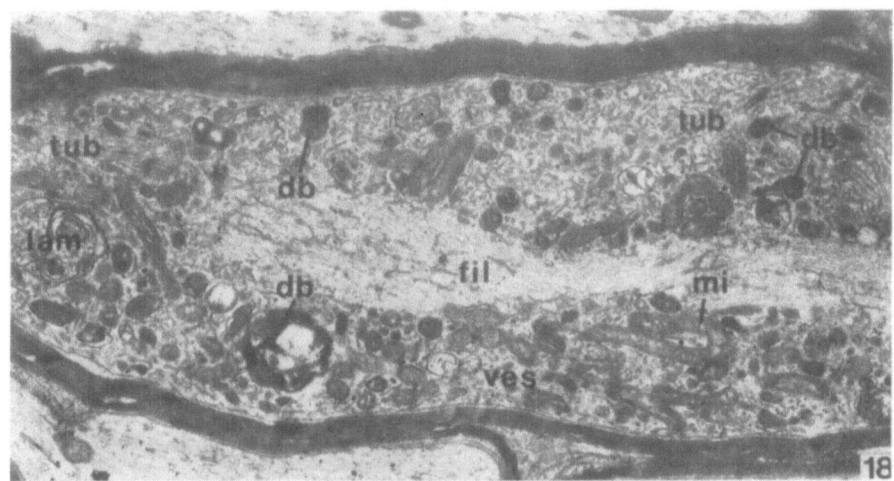

Fig. 18. 3 days at operation, 14 days survival. Longitudinal section. Part of a dilated, myelinated axon. A central core of filaments (*fil*) is surrounded by numerous mitochondria, tubular structures (*tub*), dense bodies (*db*) and vesicular profiles (*ves*). In addition, occasional lamellated bodies (*lam*) can be seen. Note the variation in the orientation and the shape of the mitochondria. One mitochondrion is u-shaped (*mi*). × 14200

into an "empty" space (Fig. 23). The cytoplasm had a lower electron density than the nucleus (Figs. 19, 20, 21, 22a and 23). Scattered groups of ribosomes, sparse endoplasmic reticulum (Figs. 19, 20, 21, 22a and b), a prominent Golgi apparatus, elongated mitochondria with clearly visible cristae (Figs. 20, 21 and 22a), lipid droplets, dense bodies and membrane-bounded bodies (see below) were usually found in the cytoplasm. Less consistent features were microtubules (cf. Fig. 24), unusual-looking mitochondria (Fig. 20) and smooth membranes of an unknown nature (see below).

The myelin-covered microglial cells regularly contained membrane-bounded bodies ranging in diameter from about 0.5–4.0 μm, the majority being 0.5 to 2.0 μm in diameter. They were bordered by one single (Fig. 27) or two unit membranes (Fig. 33). The shape of the bodies was irregular or round and their internal structure showed considerable variation. In some cases they contained a generally electron-dense matrix, in which small vesiculated parts and rounded dense profiles similar in size to mitochondria could be seen (Fig. 27). In other cases there was a granular and vesiculated matrix (Fig. 24). In yet other cases

Fig. 16. 17 days at operation, 10 days survival. Longitudinal section. Two myelin bodies; the lower one is only partially in the picture. Between the myelin layers is disintegrated cytoplasmic-like material. Above, the most peripherally situated cytoplasmic-like rim in the myelin body seems to be continuous with glial cytoplasm (*gl*) separating the myelin lamellae. × 9800. Inset: Higher magnification picture of rectangular area in Fig. 16. In most places the myelin period is normal (arrowheads). × 140000

Fig. 17. 5 days at operation, 8 days survival. Longitudinal section. Normal-looking oligo-dendrocyte surrounded by thick myelin, which at the bottom of the picture shows some bulging. Note characteristic rough-surfaced endoplasmic reticulum (*er*). × 10650

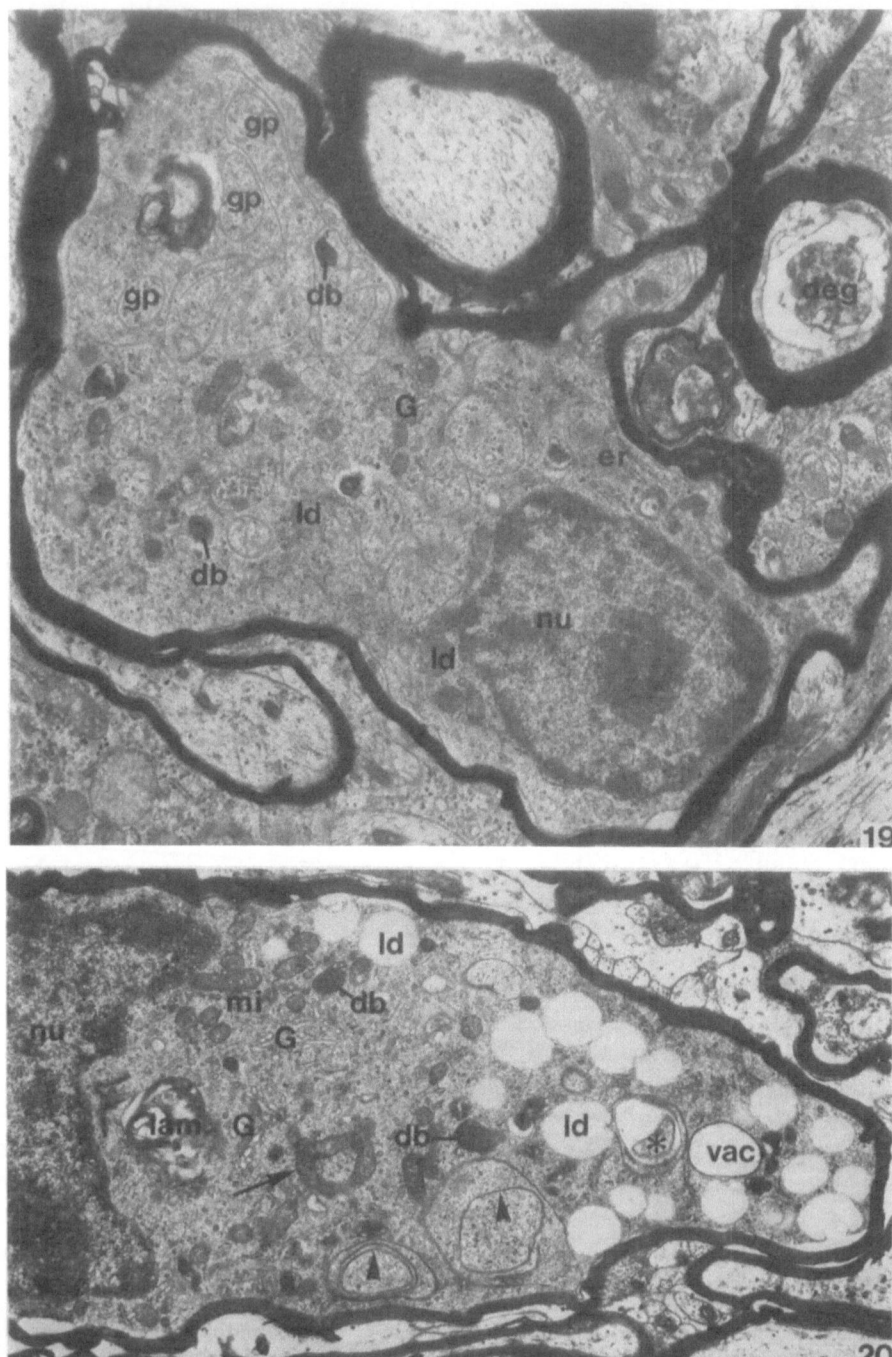

Fig. 19. 6 days at operation, 7 days survival. Transverse section. Myelincovered microglial cell. The nucleus (*nu*) is rather electron-dense with clumps of chromatin beneath the nuclear membrane. The cytoplasm is of moderate electron density. It is rather abundant and gives off processes (*gp*) which in many places invaginate the parent cell body. Groups of ribosomes

membrane-bounded formations containing vesicles and/or osmiophilic profiles
were observed in the bodies (Fig. 24). Membrane-bounded bodies having a lamellated structure were common (Fig. 23). Vacuolated parts usually occurred within
them (Figs. 23 and 29). Close examination of these bodies showed as a rule a
repeating period of 40–50 Å (Fig. 30) although in some the lamellae had a
repeating period of about 100 Å. In still others a compact appearance of the
lamellated body was noted. The lamellated bodies were sometimes associated with
lipid droplets. Many membrane-bounded bodies contained predominantly cell
organelles which seemed to be either in a normal or degenerated state. Thus,
swollen mitochondria and mitochondria with vesiculation of the cristae (Fig. 32),
clusters of ribosome-like particles (Fig. 31) and sometimes in addition mitochondria, vesicular profiles and lipid droplets (Fig. 33) were seen. Occasionally
rounded, large, dense bodies containing paracrystalline-like formations were
observed (Fig. 28). Finally a great number of membrane-bounded bodies contained
flocculent material in which unidentifiable membranous remnants occurred.

Usually the myelin-covered microglial cells filled practically the whole space
bordered by myelin (Figs. 19, 20, 22a and b), leaving in some cases only a thin
electron-lucent region next to the innermost myelin lamellae, although in a few
cases this region was considerably larger (Fig. 23). Infrequently, one or more
electron-lucent membrane-bounded formations containing granules, remnants of
membranes and sometimes also a few paracrystalline-like structures were noted in
the region between the glial cell and its myelin covering. The nature of these
areas could not be established. In no case was normal axoplasm, electron-dense
axoplasm, electron-lucent axoplasm or filamentous axoplasm seen in this region.

In some instances microglial cell processes were seen lying across the glial
cytoplasmic (terminal) pockets of a node of Ranvier (Figs. 25 and 26). At such
places the node appeared dilated (Fig. 25). Sometimes a parent cell body of at least
one of these processes could be traced and it was then always found lying outside
the myelin sheath (cf. Fig. 25). Examination of serial sections through these nodes
only rarely revealed an axon or axon-like structure within them. When found
it was tightly packed with filaments and/or partially vesiculated (Fig. 26).

In animals with survival times of 14–18 days a few atypical myelin-covered
microglial cells were observed. Their cytoplasm was to a large extent vacuolated
and filled with various membrane-bounded bodies composed of lamellated struc-

lie scattered in the cytoplasm, rough-surfaced endoplasmic reticulum (er) is poorly developed,
as is in this case also the Golgi apparatus (G). A few dense bodies (db) and lipid droplets (ld)
can be seen. The surrounding myelin appears normal. To the right a degenerating nerve
fibre (deg). × 12000

Fig. 20. 3 days at operation, 14 days survival. Longitudinal section. Myelin-covered microglial
cell. The electron-dense nucleus (nu) with clumps of chromatin is partially visible. The cytoplasm is abundant and is of moderate electron density. There are numerous lipid droplets (ld),
mitochondria (mi) and dense bodies (db). The mitochondrial cristae are often distinct. One
mitochondrion forms a ring (arrow). The Golgi apparatus (G) is prominent. Note layers of
glial processes which are wrapped around each other (arrowheads). To the right a vacuole
(vac) bordered by two unit membranes. Adjacent to these is a glial process (*) surrounded
by an empty area. A lamellar formation (lam) can be seen. The myelin covering the cell
appears normal. × 9800

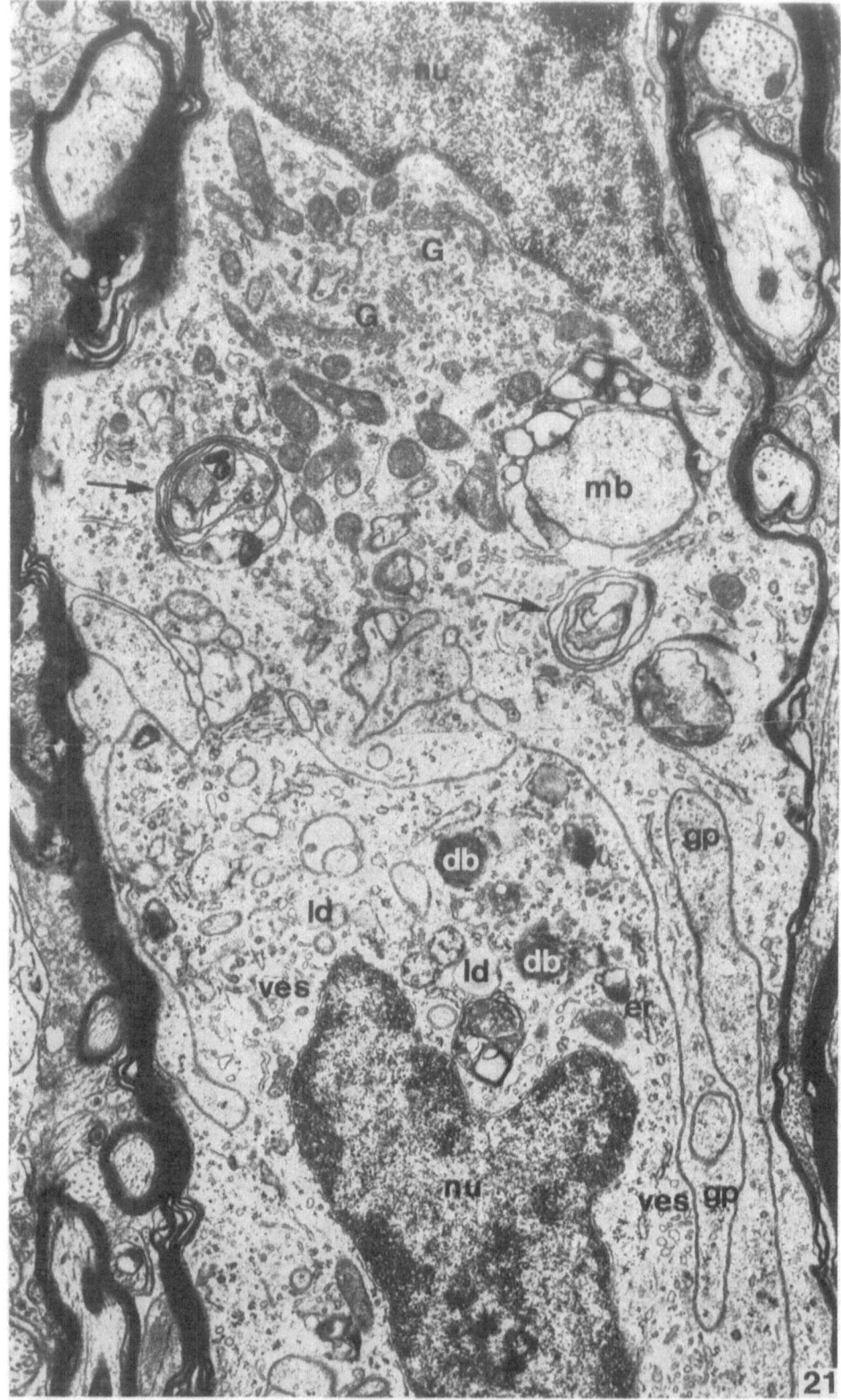

Fig. 21

tures, unidentifiable membranous formations, ribosome-like particles or dense material (Fig. 35). The nucleus of these cells had an evenly dispersed chromatin and a nuclear membrane which could be identified only at certain places around the nucleus (Fig. 35).

Degenerating Glial Cells

Structures interpreted as degenerating glial cells constituted an important feature of the process of degeneration. The majority were surrounded by myelin, but a few were situated outside myelin. A pyknotic nucleus and disorganized cytoplasm characterized the latter cells which closely resembled the degenerating glial cells found in control material. No apparent increase in the proportion of degenerating glial cells outside myelin was observed in material taken from the operated side, as compared with contralateral side or with the control material.

Degenerating cells surrounded by myelin were first seen 8 days after the operation but were rare at that time. From 9 days on, however, until about 21 days postoperatively they were common; between about 3 weeks and 2 months they were seen only occasionally. One or rarely two large (2–5 μm) electron-dense round, oval or slightly irregular bodies were consistent features of these cells (Figs. 36 and 37). Occasionally a double membrane was seen around a part of such a dense body (Fig. 36). Cells thought to be at an early stage of the degenerative process exhibited a general granular appearance (Fig. 36). Swollen mitochondria were observed in some cases. In others cases shrunken profiles, possibly mitochondria, were seen together with vacuoles and lamellated structures, which displayed the normal myelin period (Fig. 36) or a repeating period of 40–50 Å. Other cells, interpreted as being in a more advanced state of degeneration showed disrupted membranes, lipid droplets, dense vacuolated bodies and lamellated bodies. Sometimes these last appeared continuous with the surrounding myelin (Fig. 36). Frequently rings of membranes which surrounded or were themselves coated with ribosome-sized granules were observed (Fig. 37). Some degenerating cells showed practically complete disintegration of the structures outside the large dense body(ies) in that only disrupted membranes and granules of different sizes were found.

The myelin covering the degenerating glial cells appeared normal in many instances (Fig. 37). The myelin around cells interpreted as being in an advanced state of degeneration often showed loosening of its lamellae, varied in thickness and was even absent in places. Serial sections through some cells interpreted as being at a less advanced state of degeneration showed them to be completely ensheathed by myelin.

Fig. 21. 21 days at operation, 6 days survival. Longitudinal section. Parts of two microglial cells enclosed by the same myelin covering. Both cells have an electron-dense nucleus (*nu*) and considerably lighter cytoplasm. Note glial processes (*gp*) invaginating the neighbouring cell. In the cytoplasm of the cell at the top of the picture there are numerous mitochondria, some of them have distinct cristae. Golgi apparatus (*G*) is prominent. Two lamellar formations are seen (arrows) which may be glial processes layered around a granular profile. A large, granular and vacuolated body (*mb*) can be seen. In the cytoplasm of the cell below there are a few dense bodies (*db*), lipid droplets (*ld*) and numerous vesicular profiles (*ves*).
× 12000

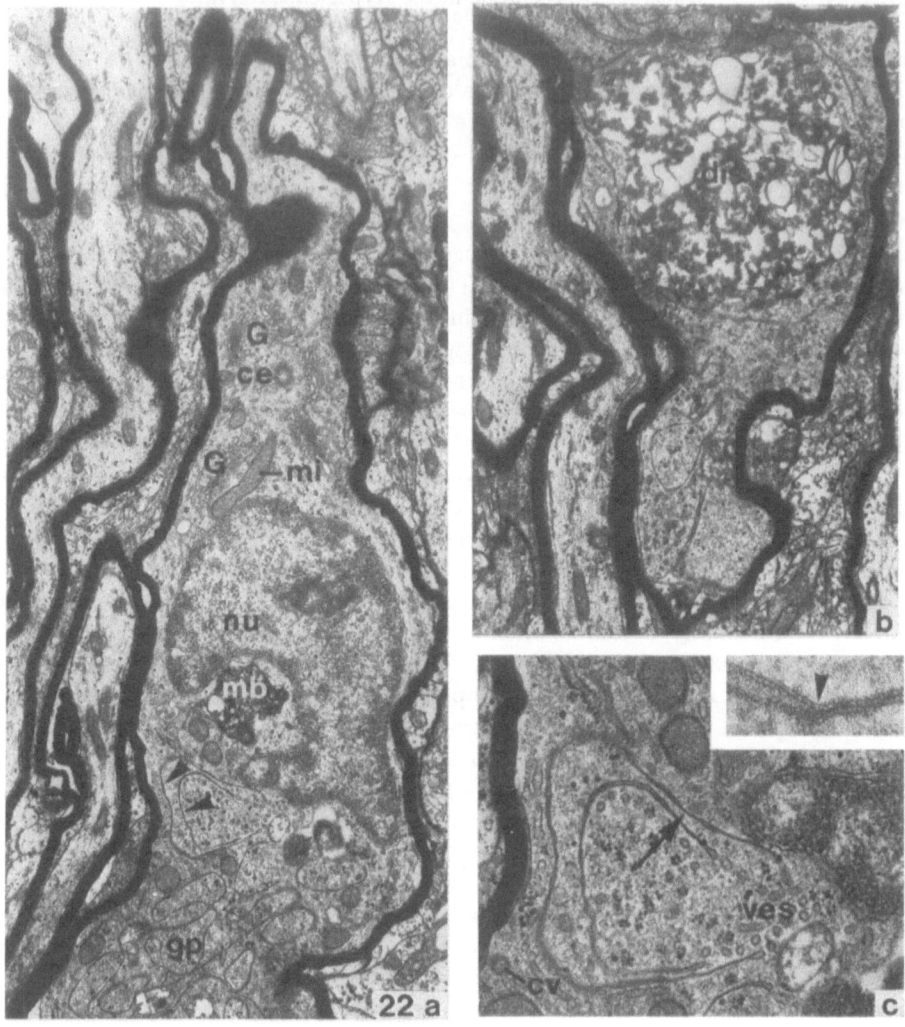

Fig. 22a—c. 6 days at operation, 5 days survival. Longitudinal section. Myelin -covered microglial cell. a Part of a myelin-covered microglial cell, the rest of which is shown in Fig. 22b. The nucleus (*nu*) is irregularly outlined and has clumps of chromatin. In the somewhat lighter cytoplasm there is a prominent Golgi apparatus (*G*), mitochondria with well defined cristae (*mi*), one centriole (*ce*), one membrane-bounded body (*mb*) with an electron-dense and vesicular content. Several processes (*gp*) extend from the cell body, some of them invaginating the cytoplasm. Close to the nucleus are a couple of intracellular membranes (arrowheads). The myelin covering the cell appears normal. × 10000. b Same section as in Fig. 22a, showing the remainder of the cell illustrated there. Note large, partially membrane-bounded formation (*dis*) containing dense structures, vacuolated areas and membranous remnants. × 10000. c Higher magnification picture of the intracellular membranes indicated by arrowheads in Fig. 22a. The membranes are seen to originate from vesicles, which seem to belong to a group of vesicular and tubular structures (*ves*), probably smooth endoplasmic reticulum or Golgi apparatus. At some places the two unit membranes come into close contact (arrow). Note coated vesicle (*cv*). × 24000. Inset: Higher magnification picture of an area of contact of the type shown at arrow in Fig. 22c. Note that the two unit membranes seemingly fuse in one place to form a fivelayered membrane complex (arrowhead). × 140000

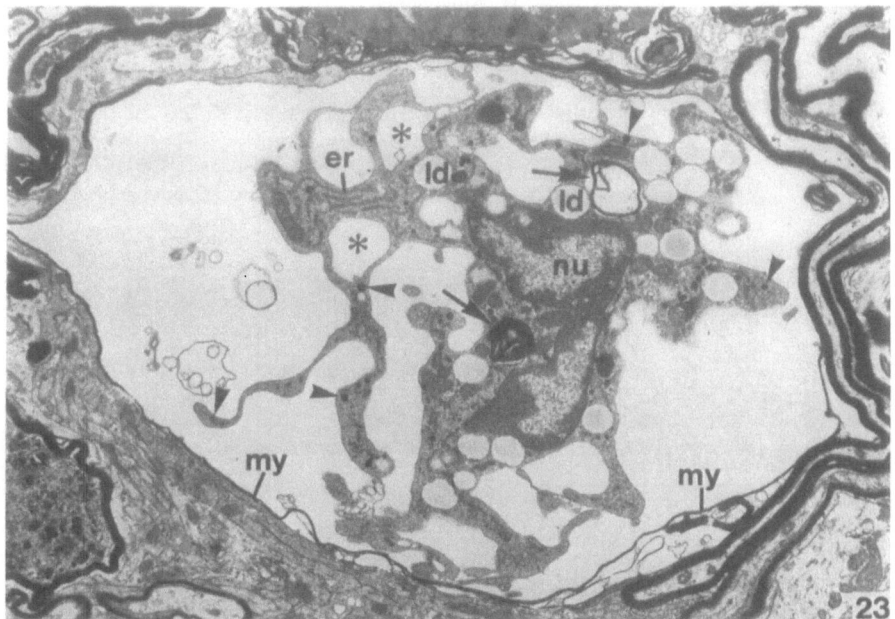

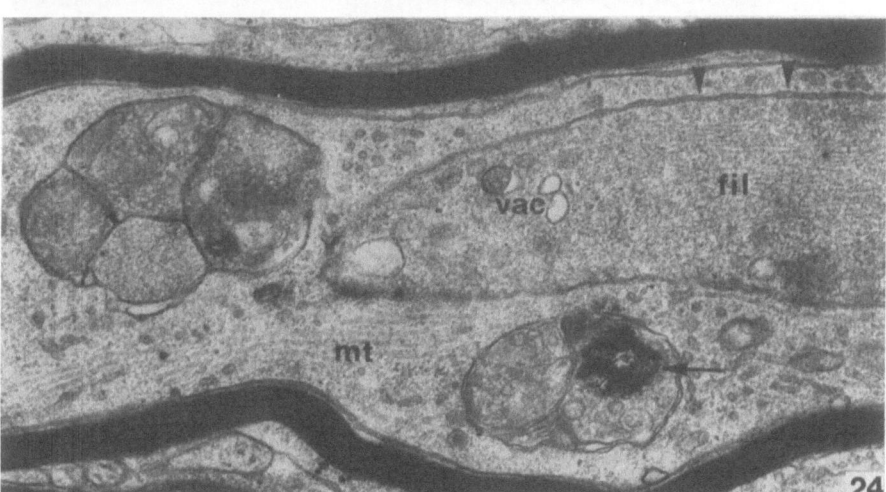

Fig. 23. 7 days at operation, 18 days survival. Longitudinal section. Microglial cell surrounded by a large "empty" space which in turn is partially bordered by thin myelin (*my*). The nucleus (*nu*) is indented and has conspicuous condensations of chromatin beneath the nuclear membrane. In the moderately electron-dense cytoplasm are numerous lipid droplets (*ld*) and dense bodies, some of which are very small (arrowheads). Two membrane-bounded lamellar bodies are seen (arrows). The rough-surfaced endoplasmic reticulum (*er*) is rather well developed for this type of cell. Several slender glial processes extend into the "empty" space. Some of these are fenestrated (*). × 5 600

Fig. 24. 17 days at operation, 10 days survival. Longitudinal section. Part of a process, probably belonging to a microglial cell. Longitudinally running microtubules (*mt*) are visible in the cytoplasm of the process. To the right part of an axon with tightly packed filaments (*fil*) and vacuoles (*vac*). There seem to be two unit membranes around the axon (arrowheads). In addition two membrane-bounded bodies can be seen in the glial process. The one on the left consists of four separate compartments which have a granular appearance. That on the right consists of two separate portions, both of which have a granular and vesicular appearance. In one of them there is in addition a highly osmiophilic structure (arrow). × 27 500

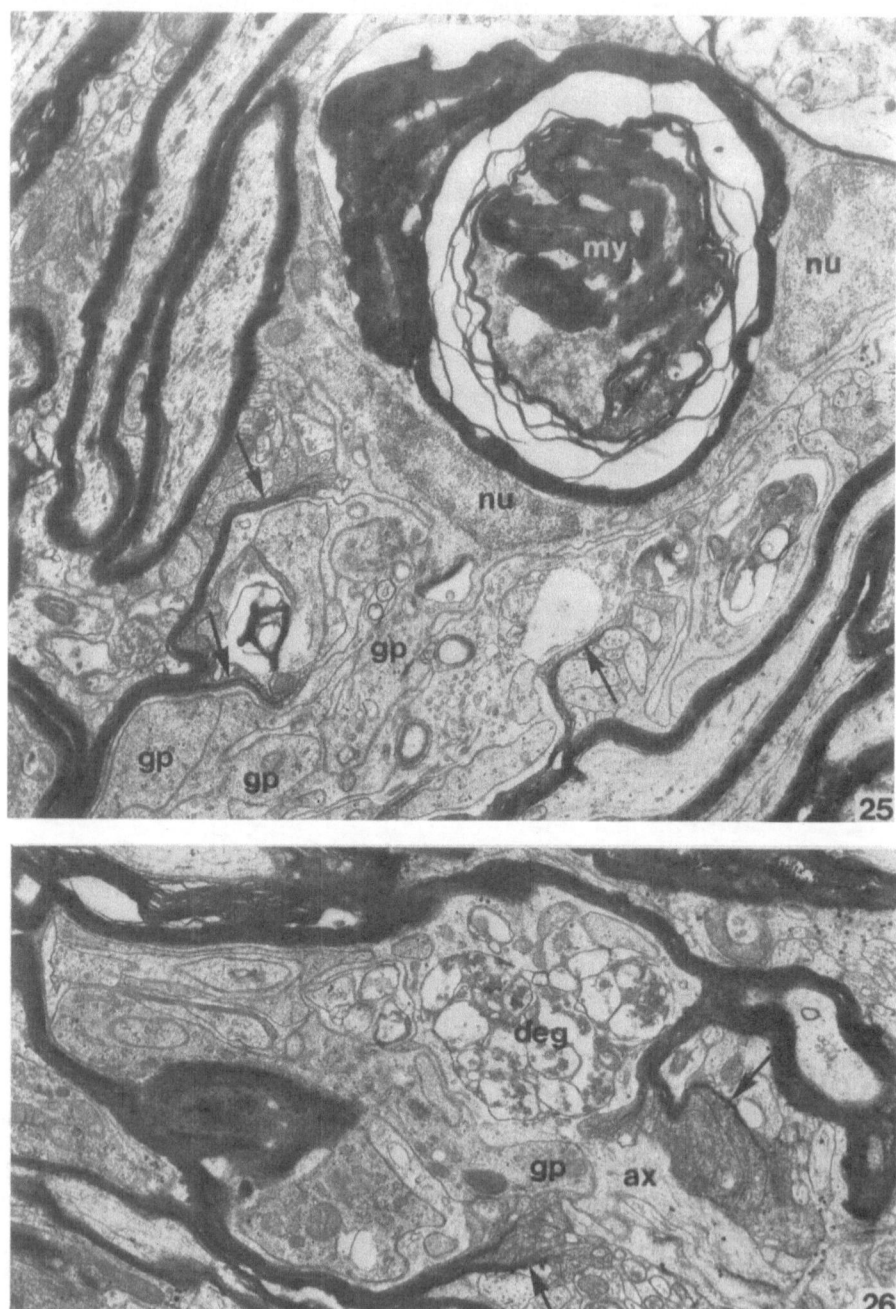

Fig. 25. 17 days at operation, 10 days survival. Longitudinal section. A dilated node of Ranvier. The splitting up of some of the myelin lamellae from an internodal segment is seen (arrows). At the node several microglial cell processes (gp) can be seen, one of which emerges from the cell body of a microglial cell (nucleus = nu) enclosing a fragment of a degenerating fibre (my). No axon can be seen in the picture. × 12000

Microglial Cells (Outside Myelin)

An increase in the number of microglial cells located outside myelin was evident from 9 days postoperatively onwards (cf. Diagram 1), the largest number being seen at about 2–3 weeks. These cells had an irregular and, in sections cut longitudinally to the root fibres, an elongated outline (Figs. 38 and 39). The nucleus was irregular, electron-dense and showed patches of chromatin adjacent to the nuclear membrane (Figs. 38, 39 and 40). The cytoplasm was less electron-dense than the nucleus (Figs. 38 and 39). Sparse endoplasmic reticulum, scattered groups of ribosomes, mitochondria with distinct cristae, narrow Golgi cisterns (Fig. 38), dense bodies and lipid droplets were common features of the cytoplasm of these cells (Figs. 38 and 39).

The vast majority of these cells contained phagocytosed degenerating structures (Figs. 38, 39 and 40). Most frequently these structures had a lamellated configuration with a repeating period of 40–50 Å (Fig. 38). Crystal-like inclusions were rarely observed in microglial cells. Occasionally myelin-covered, electron-dense axoplasmic fragments (Fig. 39) or degenerating glial cells (Fig. 40) were found to have been phagocytosed by microglial cells.

Pericytes

At 21 to 35 days postoperatively the incidence of pericytes containing vacuoles and dense bodies was increased. Some pericytes were heavily loaded with such structures (Fig. 41), a feature not encountered in the normal material. Lamellated structures electron-dense axoplasmic fragments or degenerating glial cells were not found in any perivascular cell. No pictures were seen suggesting a migration of cells through the basement membrane either into or from the interstitial space nor were any pictures obtained suggesting cell migration through the vessel wall.

Mitotic cells

Mitotic cells were observed more frequently than in the control material or than in experimental material taken from the unoperated side. Most of these cells occurred from 1 to 2 weeks postoperatively. It was not possible to classify them. Two mitotic cells were observed to contain degenerating nerve fibre fragments, lipid droplets and dense bodies (Fig. 42).

Oligodendrocytes

Between 25 and 35 days postoperatively a few oligodendrocytes were seen ensheathed by a couple of myelin lamellae (Fig. 43). It was not established whether this myelin covered the glial cells completely or not. No morphological changes were observed in the oligodendrocytes.

Fig. 26. 17 days at operation, 10 days survival. Longitudinal section. A dilated node of Ranvier. The splitting up of the myelin lamellae and the glial cytoplasmic (terminal) pockets (arrows) is visible. A microglial cell process (gp) is seen, adjacent to some of the terminal pockets. The axon (ax) seems to be constricted and a great part of its internodal portion has a vesicular appearance (deg). × 12250

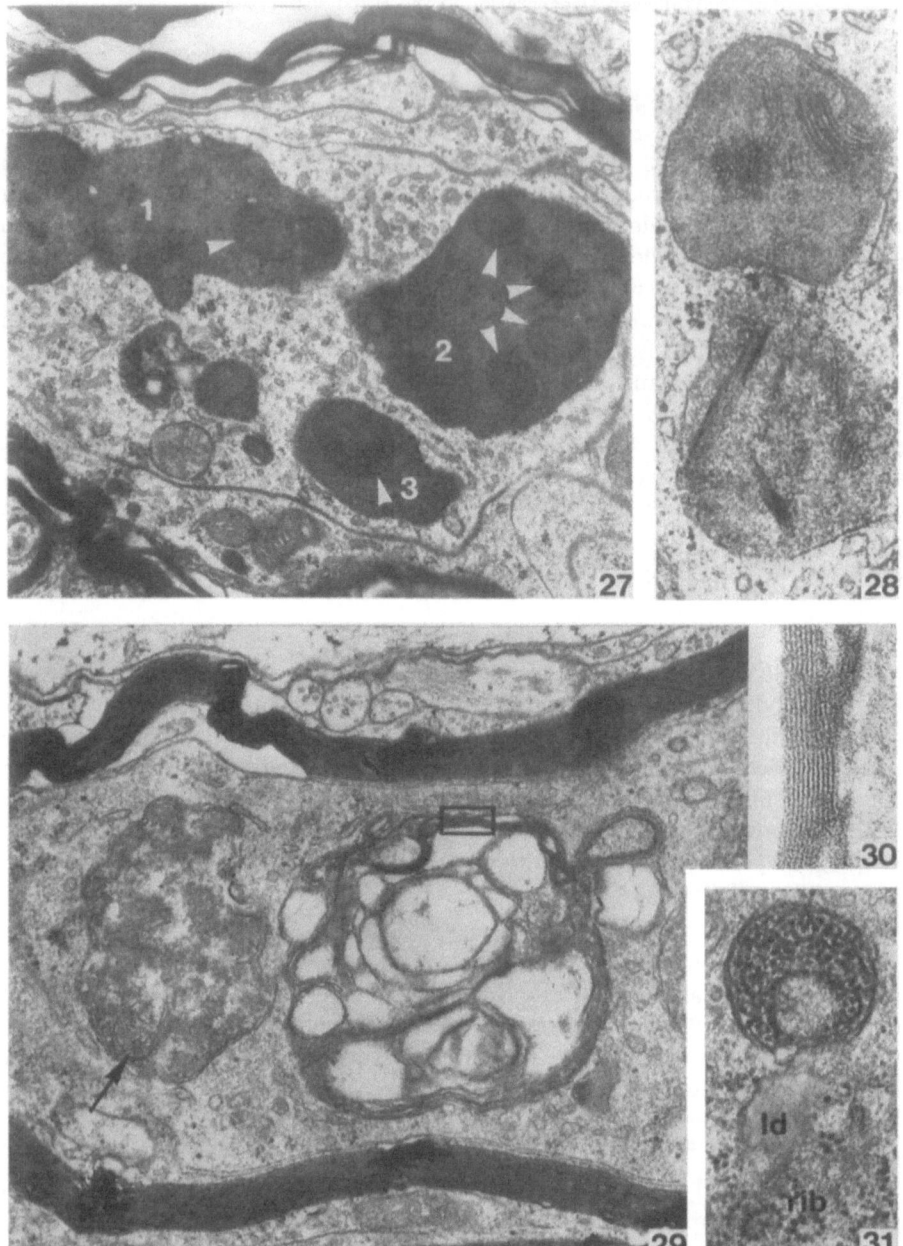

Fig. 27. 25 days at operation, 12 days survival. Longitudinal section. Part of a myelin-covered microglial cell enclosing three membrane-bounded bodies (*1, 2* and *3*) with electron-dense matrix. A few vesicular areas can be seen in *1*. In addition there are several electron-dense, rounded structures (arrowheads), similar in size to mitochondria. × 16 500

Fig. 28. 6 days at operation, 5 days survival. Part of a myelin-covered microglial cell with two membrane-bounded bodies having a dense matrix containing a few paracrystalline-like structures. × 44 000

Fig. 29. 2 days at operation, 7 days survival. Longitudinal section. Part of a myelin-covered microglial cell with two membrane-bounded bodies. The one on the left has areas of alternating high and low electron density and contains a structure (arrow) which may be a mitochondrion. That on the right has a mainly lamellated configuration. × 28 400

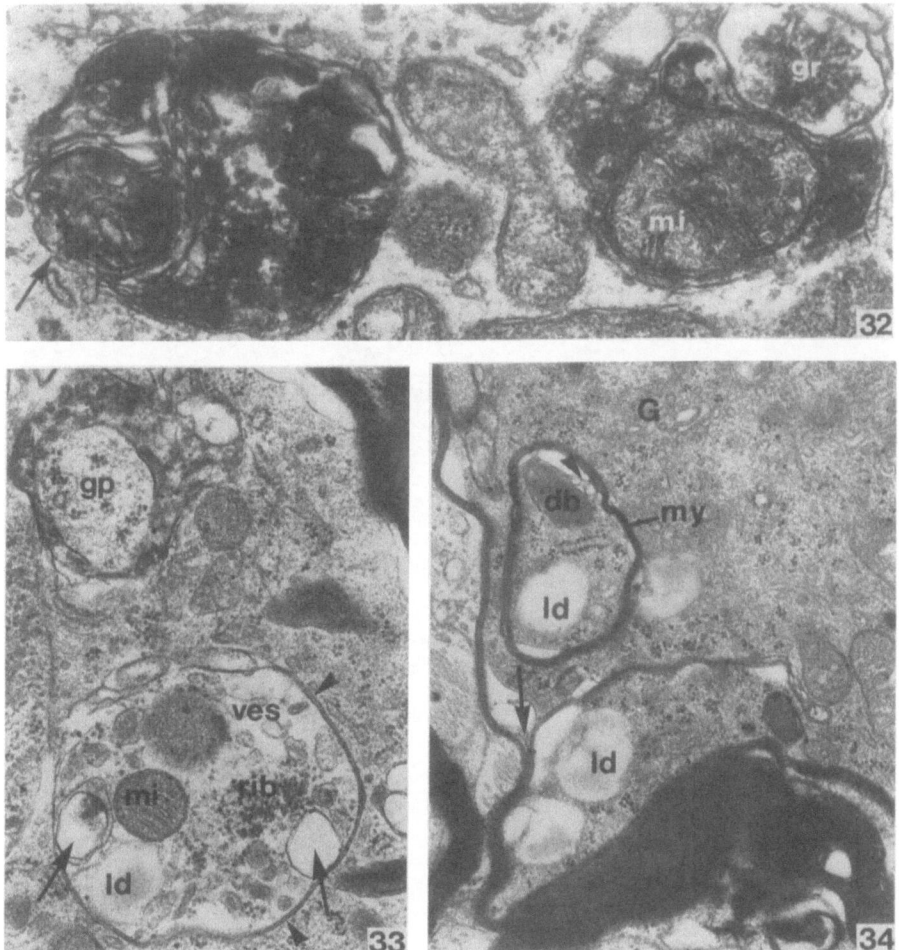

Fig. 32. 21 days at operation, 6 days survival. Two membrane-bounded bodies with mainly electron-dense matrix. The one on the left contains what is probably a mitochondrion (arrow) with vesiculated cristae. That on the right contains a swollen mitochondrion (*mi*) in which only few cristae are intact. Adjacent to this last body is a membrane-bounded structure with a granular content (*gr*). Note single unit membrane bordering the membrane-bounded bodies.
× 44000

Fig. 33. 2 days at operation, 7 days survival. Above, a dense partially vacuolated structure penetrated by a glial process (*gp*). Below, a membrane-bounded body containing one normal-looking mitochondrion (*mi*), a few vesicular structures (*ves*), two vacuoles (arrows), one lipid droplet (*ld*) and a group of ribosome-sized particles (*rib*). Note the two unit membranes bordering the body (arrowheads). × 27000

Fig. 34. 6 days at operation, 7 days survival. Transverse section. Part of a myelin-covered microglial cell. The cell is covered by myelin which is partially detached (arrow). Note the ring of myelin (*my*) which is connected with a dense body (*db*) by short bridges (arrowhead). In the cytoplasm can be seen Golgi apparatus (*G*) and lipid droplets (*ld*). × 22000

Fig. 30. Higher magnification picture of rectangular area in Fig. 29. Note uniform lamellar period of the order of 40–50 Å. × 140000

Fig. 31. 2 days at operation, 7 days survival. Above, membrane-bounded body containing a great number of closely packed ribosome-sized granules. In the surrounding cytoplasm several ribosomes (*rib*) can be seen and one lipid droplet (*ld*). × 45000

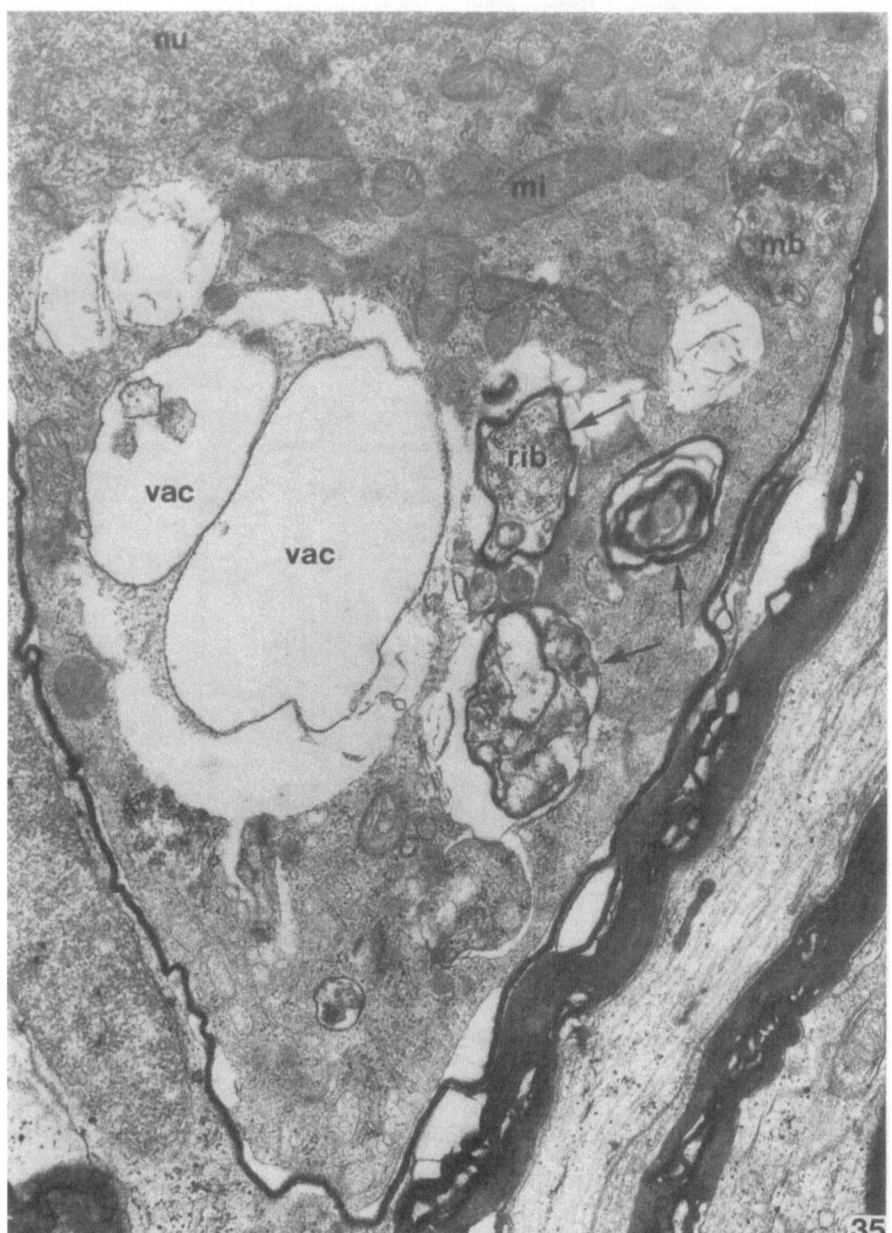

Fig. 35. 5 days at operation, 15 days survival. Longitudinal section. Part of a myelin-covered microglial cell (nucleus = nu). The nuclear membrane is poorly outlined. The cytoplasm is characterized by two large vacuoles (vac) and several membrane-bounded bodies. Three of them have a lamellated content (arrows).   In one of these three bodies there are in addition numerous ribosome-sized particles (rib). A fourth membrane-bounded body (mb) contains unidentifiable membranous formations and ribosome-sized particles. Note that the ribosomes in the cytoplasm show little tendency to polysome formation. × 14200

Fig. 36. 6 days at operation, 18 days survival. Longitudinal section. Degenerating glial cell covered by myelin. The pyknotic nucleus (py) is surrounded by remnants of the nuclear membrane (arrowhead). The cytoplasm has a granular appearance and contains several small medium-dense profiles, which may be shrunken mitochondria. In addition there are two lamellated structures (lam). The one on the right is continuous with the myelin surrounding

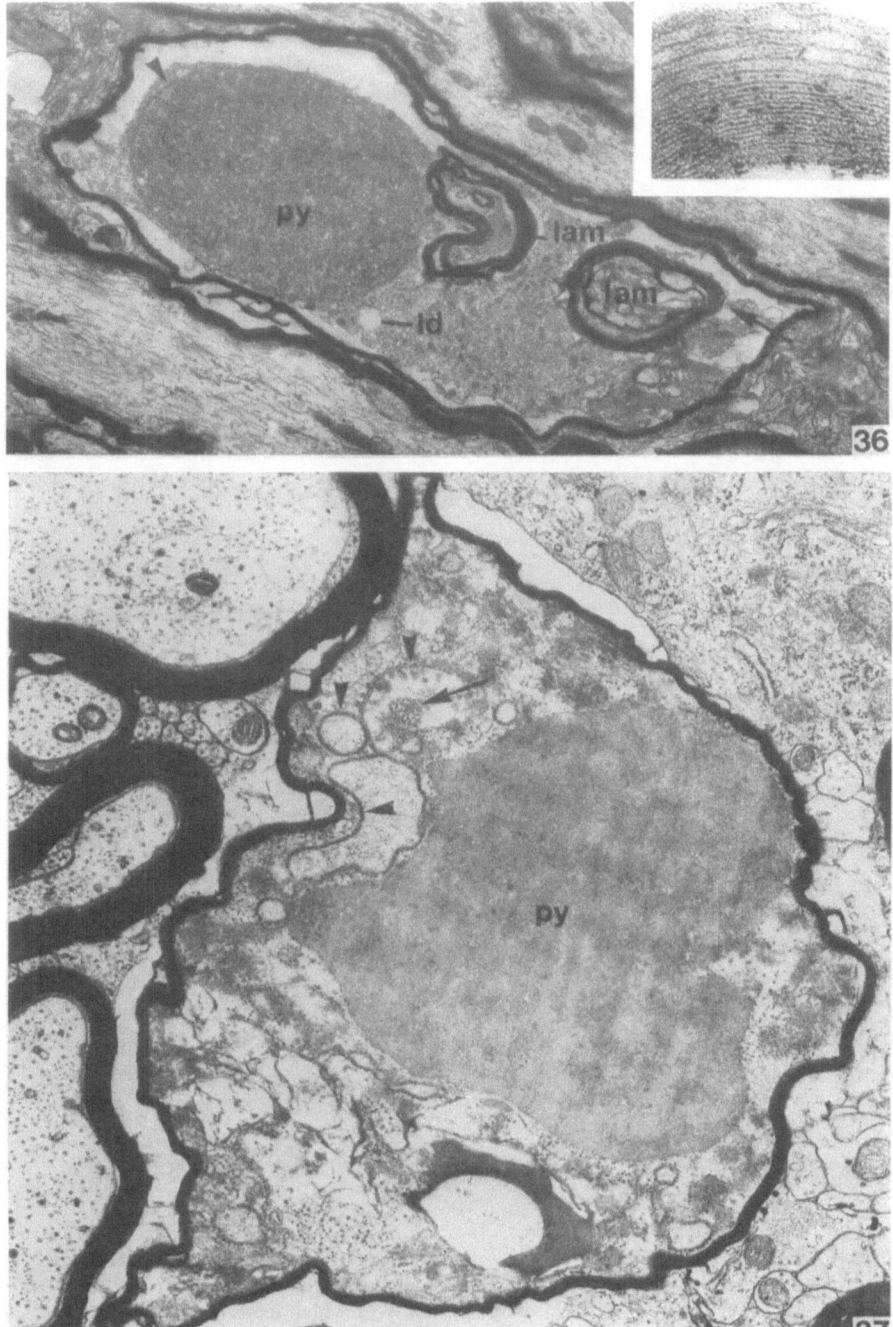

the degenerating cell. × 12250. Inset: Higher magnification picture of the part of the lamellated structure in Fig. 36 labelled with an arrow. A myelin-like appearance of the lamellated structure is evident. × 90000

Fig. 37. 15 days at operation, 15 days survival. Transverse section. Degenerating glial cell covered by normal-looking myelin. The cell is characterized by a pyknotic nucleus (*py*) and completely disorganized cytoplasm. Rings of membranes coated with ribosome-sized particles are seen (arrowheads). In addition a cluster of ribosome-sized particles can be seen (arrow). × 21000

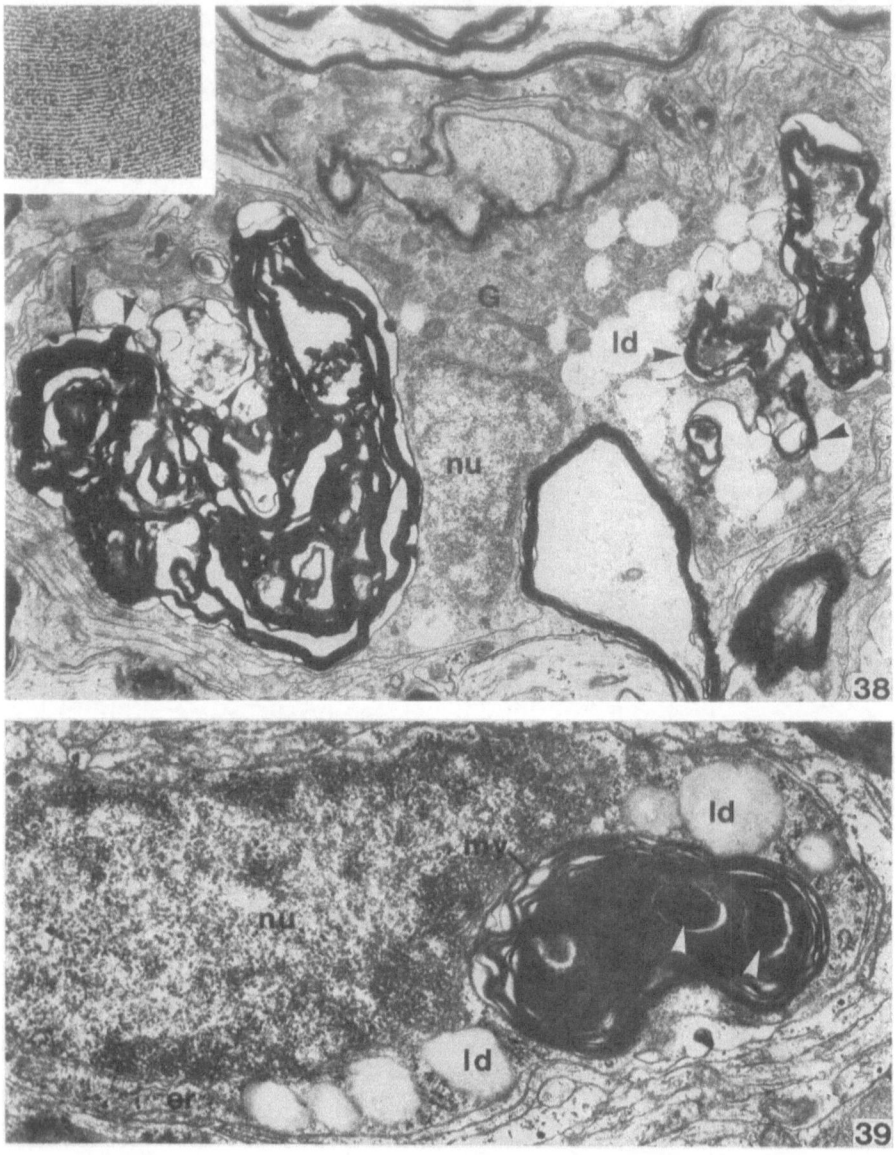

Fig. 38. 7 days at operation, 18 days survival. Longitudinal section. Microglial cell (nucleus = *nu*) with two large inclusions consisting primarily of lamellar structures. In the cytoplasm are a large number of lipid droplets, many of which seem to be directly associated with the lamellar inclusions (arrowheads). The Golgi apparatus (*G*) consists of several narrow cisterns. × 10000. Inset: Higher magnification picture of the part of the lamellar structure labelled with arrow. It shows a uniform repeating period of about 50 Å. × 135000

Fig. 39. 25 days at operation, 9 days survival. Longitudinal section. Microglial cell with a phagocytosed fragment of an electron-dense myelinated axon. The myelin lamellae (*my*) are loosely arranged. In the dense axoplasm two rounded structures (arrowheads), probably mitochondria, are seen. The nucleus (*nu*) of the glial cell has clumps of chromatin beneath the nuclear membrane. The cytoplasm contains several lipid droplets (*ld*), scattered groups of ribosomes and a few membranes of rough-surfaced endoplasmic reticulum (*er*). × 18000

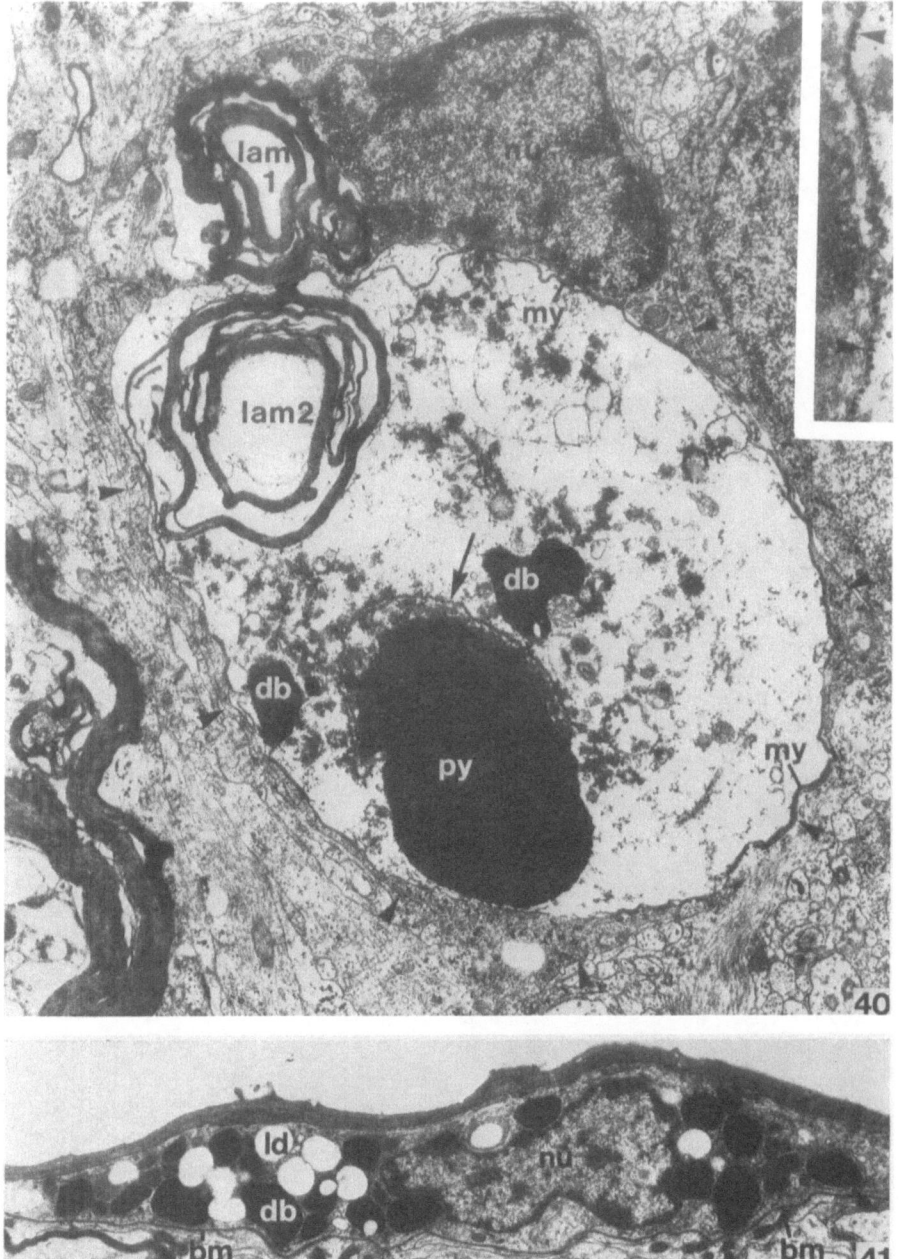

Fig. 40. 6 days at operation, 9 days survival. Longitudinal section. A microglial cell with characteristic nucleus (*nu*) showing high electron density and conspicuous clumping of chromatin. The scanty cytoplasm, the periphery of which is labelled with arrowheads, contains a lamellar structure (*lam 1*) and a structure interpreted as the remains of a degenerating glial cell. The latter is partially surrounded by thin myelin (*my*) which is continuous with a lamellar structure (*lam 2*). Associated with what is probably the pyknotic nucleus (*py*) is a membranous remnant (arrow). × 12000. Inset: Higher magnification picture of area close to arrow in Fig. 40. It can be seen that the membrane is coated with ribosome-sized particles. × 42000

Fig. 41. 6 days at operation, 35 days survival. Longitudinal section. Pericyte (nucleus = *nu*) within basement membrane (*bm*). The cytoplasm is loaded with dense bodies (*db*), and lipid droplets (*ld*). × 5600

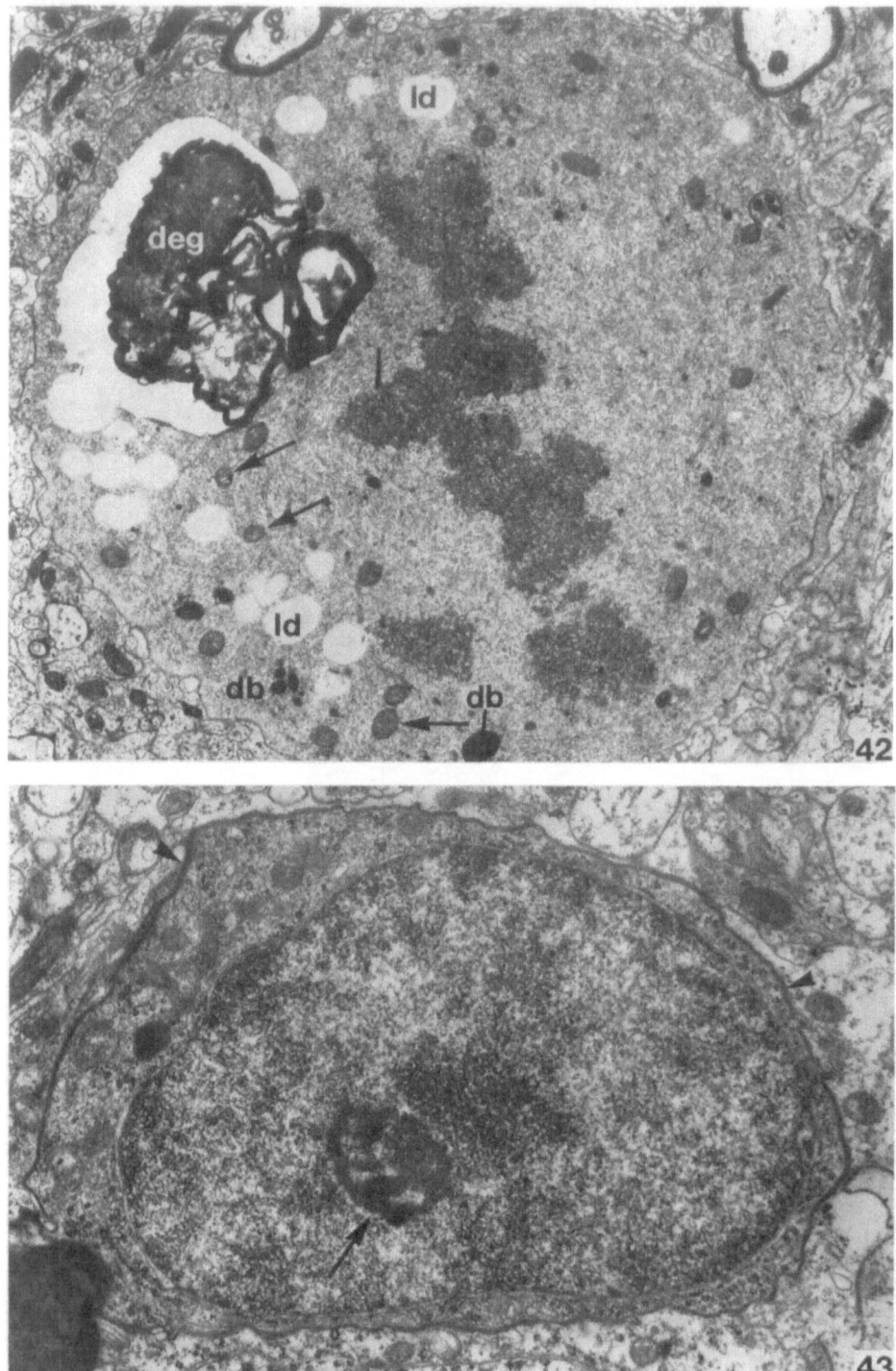

Figs. 42 and 43

Astrocytes

From 25 days onwards hypertrophic astrocytes were observed and by 60 days these were numerous. The cytoplasm of these astrocytes was abundant and rich in organelles (Fig. 44). An increase over normal was apparent in the amount of endoplasmic reticulum, Golgi cisterns, dense bodies, gliosomes and filaments (Fig. 44). Microtubules, rarely encountered in the astrocytes of the control material were regularly found in the hypertrophic astrocytes (Figs. 44 and 45). A large increase in the number of astrocytic cell processes filled with filaments was evident (although the actual number of astrocytes did not seem to have changed) forming a glial scar (Fig. 43). There was no detectable increase in the number of glycogen granules in these processes. The astrocytes did not show any signs of phagocytic activity.

γ) **Comparison of Results Obtained from Animals Operated on at Different Ages.** Two differences were observed when comparing the process of fibre degeneration in the three groups of kittens (cf. Table 1). Firstly the numbers of degenerating nerve fibres seemed to be considerably less in groups II (10 to 17 days) and III (21 to 28 days) than in group I (2 to 7 days). This was particularly striking when groups III and I were compared. Secondly, the process of degeneration seemed to manifest itself somewhat earlier in group I than in groups II and III e.g. electron-dense axons were first seen at 3, 5 and 6 days in group I, II and III respectively. The type of changes observed were qualitatively the same as those described for the youngest group (I) in the two older groups of kittens.

IV. Discussion

Possible Errors in the Interpretation of the Experimental Findings

It is important to consider the possibility that the changes observed here might have been influenced or caused by factors other than the transection of the nerve. Two such possible factors are: preparatory artifacts and "spontaneous" degeneration.

Preparatory artifacts are considered unlikely as the cause of the principle changes observed here, for the following reasons. The changes described here occurred in regions which, according to currently standard criteria (see e.g. Hayat, 1970) were well preserved. They occurred either selectively on the operated side or increased significantly on that side. The degenerative changes were accompanied by a glial cell reaction involving both phagocytosis of degenerating structures and formation of a glial scar.

Fig. 42. 7 days at operation, 21 days survival. Longitudinal section. Mitotic glial cell containing a fragment of a degenerating myelinated fibre (*deg*), several lipid droplets (*ld*) and dense bodies (*db*). The distinct appearance of the cristae of some of the mitochondria should be noted (arrows). × 9800

Fig. 43. 6 days at operation, 25 days survival. Oligodendrocyte surrounded by very thin myelin (arrowheads). Note the high electron density of both nucleus and cytoplasm, the prominent nucleolus (arrow) and the abundance of free ribosomes, all features characteristic of normal oligodendrocytes. × 14700

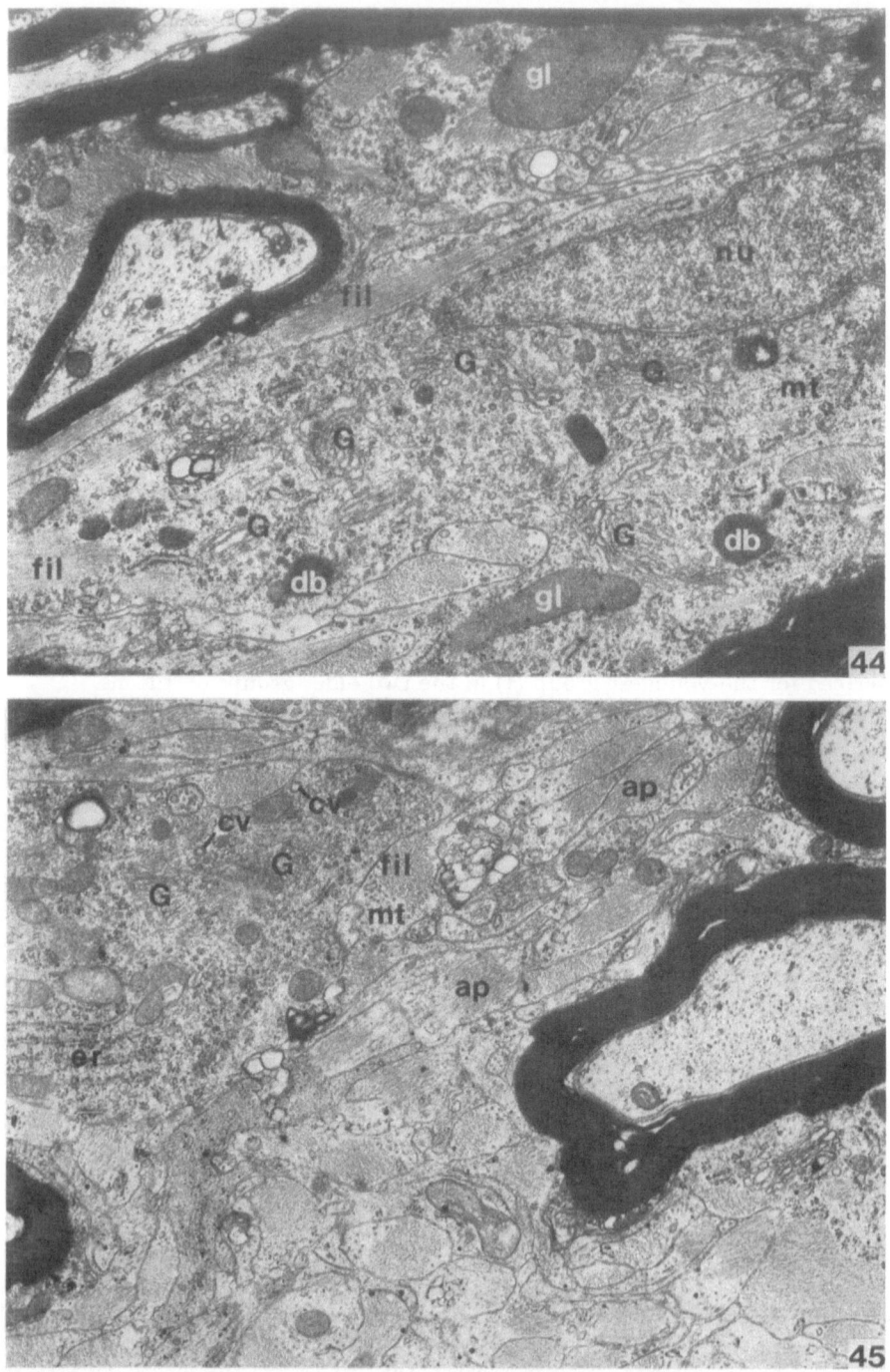

Fig. 44. 5 days at operation, 60 days survival. Longitudinal section. Part of an astrocyte
(nucleus = *nu*) with abundant, organelle-rich cytoplasm. Note prominent Golgi apparatus (*G*),
dense bodies, (*db*), filaments (*fil*) and microtubules (*mt*) in the cytoplasm. Two gliosomes (*gl*)
of moderate size are also visible. × 14 200

In material perfused with the cacodylate-buffered fixative solution extensive myelin sheath splitting was common. This was probably due to the low tonicity of the cacodylate buffer (cf. Berthold, 1968; Hildebrand, 1971a). Since other tissue components appeared adequately preserved, these animals were nevertheless, included in the material studied, but were of course not used in evaluating myelin sheath changes. In structures where disintegration of membranous components takes place it is possible that for instance osmotic changes occur which make conventionally employed fixative solutions incapable of adequate fixation. The penetration of fixatives may be impaired in regions where degeneration occurs. For these reasons it seems advisable to be very cautious in drawing conclusions about the *in vivo* situation from the experimental findings.

The existence of "spontaneous" degeneration is well established both in the central and the peripheral nervous systems. An increased incidence of such degeneration seems to occur during the postnatal development of the nervous system (Spatz, 1918; Bodian, 1966; Berthold and Skoglund, 1968a, b; Das and Hine, 1971; Hildebrand, 1971; Aguayo et al., 1973; Reier and Hughes, 1973). A careful study of control material is therefore of crucial importance. Some studies have shown that changes can take place in a nerve fibre system following a lesion of the same system on the contralateral side (Cole and Nauta, 1970; Muirhead and Mezei, 1973). Thus it seems wise to rely primarily on nonoperated material as was done here, rather than on material from the unoperated side, to obtain information about the normal appearance of the system under study.

In the control material there were signs of myelin sheath (Figs. 7, 9) and glial cell degeneration (Fig. 10). The myelin sheath changes were similar to some described by Hildebrand (1971b) in the normal kitten spinal cord. He also observed degenerating glial cells, which were considered to be oligodendrocytes. It has not been possible to establish the nature of the degenerating glial cells observed in the present study. They may be oligodendrocytes and thus possibly a reflection of a programmed cell death affecting some oligodendroglial-myelin units during postnatal development (Hildebrand, 1971b). However, evidence for glial cell degeneration in the adult central nervous system has also been presented (Pannese and Ferranini, 1967; Mori and Leblond, 1970) and proliferation of glial cells seems to occur throughout life (Smart and Leblond, 1961; Hommes and Leblond, 1967; Dalton et al., 1968). It is therefore possible that some of the degenerating glial cells found here are the products of a slow continuous degeneration of glial cells and thus not specific for the developmental period.

No conclusive pictures of degenerating axoplasm in the form of electron-dense axoplasm (see e.g. Guillery, 1970) filamentous axoplasm (Mugnaini and Walberg, 1967) or electron-lucent axoplasm (O'Neal and Westrum, 1973) were obtained in the control material. In the myelin bodies, granular or disintegrated

Fig. 45. 5 days at operation, 60 days survival. Transverse section. A great number of astrocytic processes (*ap*) occupy most of the area shown in the picture. They contain tightly packed filaments (*fil*) and in addition often a few microtubules (*mt*). To the left, part of the cytoplasm of an astrocyte with numerous free ribosomes, well-developed endoplasmic reticulum (*er*), a Golgi apparatus (*G*) and coated vesicles (*cv*). × 14200 cytoplasmic-like material was often found, however (Fig. 7). Whether this represents axoplasmic or glial cytoplasmic remnants could not be established. Therefore, the question of whether axonal degeneration occurs normally in the system studied here cannot be answered.

In summary, there was evidence for the occurrence of degenerative changes affecting some myelin sheaths and glial cells in the control material. Because of the sparseness of these degenerating structures they could constitute, however, only a small part of the degenerative changes observed after nerve transection.

The Experimentally Induced Degeneration of Myelinated Nerve Fibres

The degenerative changes in the myelinated nerve fibres appeared as electron-dense axons (Figs. 12, 14 and 15), shrunken axons (Fig. 12), myelin bodies (Figs. 12 and 16) and aberrant myelin (Figs. 11c, d and 17). These changes coincide with changes previously described for fibres undergoing Wallerian degeneration in adult animals (see e.g. Lampert and Cressman, 1966; Lampert, 1967a; McMahan, 1967; Mugnaini et al., 1967; Bignami and Ralston, 1969; Dunkerley and Duncan, 1969) and kittens (Hildebrand, 1971b; Pecci Saveedra et al., 1973).

The findings made here indicated that axonal degeneration occurs before myelin sheath degeneration. This is in agreement with most previous studies on direct Wallerian degeneration (Wechsler and Hager, 1962; Nathaniel and Pease, 1963; McMahan, 1967; Cravioto, 1969; Nathaniel and Nathaniel, 1973).

Hence the qualitative appearance and temportal sequence of the changes in myelinated nerve fibres seem to be the same during indirect Wallerian degeneration in the central nervous part of the hypoglossal nerve of the kitten as during direct Wallerian degeneration in adult mammals and kittens. It should be pointed out, however, that so far no *systematic* study has been carried out on direct Wallerian degeneration in immature animals. It remains to be shown too, whether the degenerative changes in myelinated nerve fibres described here occur during indirect Wallerian degeneration in adult animals.

The Early Reaction of Microglial Cells

Some of the most conspicuous changes in the present study concern the myelin-covered microglial cells.

The present findings indicate that these cells are as a rule completely covered with myelin. Firstly, in single sections the cells were, with few exceptions, completely covered by myelin both in sections cut transversely and longitudinally in relation to the intramedullary root fibres of the hypoglossal nerve. Secondly, examination of serial sections of some of these cells did not reveal any opening in the myelin. This relationship between myelin and glial cell may result from migration of the glial cell inside a myelin sheath, in which later on, a fusion of the proximal and distal open ends of myelin takes place. The pictures in which microglial cell processes were seen lying across the terminal pockets at a node of Ranvier (Figs. 25 and 26) suggest that this is a place where migration to its position with in the myelin sheath can take place, in a similar fashion to some of the mononuclear cells appearing in experimental allergic encephalomyelitis in the rat (Lampert, 1967b) and in experimental spongy degeneration of the rat (Lampert and Schochet, 1968). Alternatively, the myelin covering of these microglial cells may be due a process of remyelination by the glial cell itself or by another glial cell. Conceivably, the stimulus for such a process could be loss of myelin from the myelinated nerve fibres. In the present situation such loss seems to be negligible or slight at the time when myelin-covered microglial cells first occur. Furthermore, in the central nervous system remyelination appears first in the form of unusually thin myelin sheaths, whereas in the present situation, the myelin covering microglial cells usually seemed to be of normal thickness (Figs. 19, 20, 22a and b).

The myelin-covered microglial cells are in many respects similar to the microglial cells seen in the control material. It must be emphasized, however, that this does not necessarily imply that the myelin-covered microglial cells originate from the normally occurring microglial cells. It has been shown in previous studies that in association with degeneration of central nervous tissue perivascular and/or haematogenous cells may enter the central nervous system and become transformed into cells which cannot be morphologically distinguished with certainty from microglial cells (Russel, 1962; Konigsmark and Sidman, 1963; Blakemore, 1972a; Kitamura et al., 1972; Matthews and Kruger, 1973; Oehmichen et al., 1973). The present findings do not give any clue as to the origin of the myelin-covered microglial cells.

Membrane-bounded bodies were usually observed in the cytoplasm of the myelin-covered microglial cells. Possibly these bodies belong to the group of lysosomes. Histochemical studies would be necessary to test this suggestion. The appearance of some of these bodies give certain indications concerning their nature. Membrane-bounded bodies having a primarily electron-dense matrix in which mitochondria-like formations were observed (Fig. 27) is resembling axoplasm undergoing degeneration. The frequent observation that no normal or degenerating axoplasm occurred between the glial cells and the surrounding myelin, indicates that the presumed axoplasmic fragments in the glial cells had originated from the axon which once existed inside the myelin. This suggestion is further supported by pictures showing microglial cell processes inside myelin sheaths surrounding axoplasm, which was partially vesiculated and which contained tightly packed filaments (Fig. 24).

Membrane-bounded bodies of a primarily lamellated appearance (Figs. 23 and 29) may be degenerating myelin or membranous remnants of other degenerating structures. The possibility of preparatory artifacts must, however, be considered in this context. Storage of tissue in aldehyde solutions may induce the formation of so-called myelin figures (Trump and Ericsson, 1965). Lamellated bodies were observed in the present study also in material prepared within a few hours of perfusion. Hence, it seems likely that at least a large proportion of these bodies do not occur as a result of storage in the fixative. Some pictures suggest that lamellated bodies may arise from detached parts of the myelin covering of the glial cell (Fig. 34). Other pictures suggest that a microglial cell containing a phagocytosed myelin sheath fragment may migrate inside the myelin (Fig. 25). It seems, however, as if the first target of the myelin-covered microglial cell would be degenerating axoplasm. Although the axoplasm once existing inside the myelin has usually been completely removed, the myelin around the microglial cell often appears normal (Figs. 19, 20, 22a and b). Membrane-bounded bodies containing predominantly cell organelles or structures resembling cell organelles (Figs. 31, 32 and 33) may appear as a result of focal segregation of cytoplasm belonging to the glial cell itself. In this case, these bodies would belong to the class of lysosomes termed autophagosomes (DeDuve and Wattiaux, 1966). Alternatively, they might contain glial cell cytoplasm from other glial cells and thus be heterophagosomes (DeDuve and Wattiaux, 1966). This second possibility seems less likely than the first, however. The appearance of autophagosomes in myelin-covered microglial cells may indicate that such cells are under some kind of metabolic stress (cf. Daniel and Strich, 1969). Augmented autophagy often occurs in cells subjected to sublethal injury (for reviews see DeDuve and Wattiaux, 1966; Ericsson, 1969). Augmented autophagy may also develop prior to cell death (Scharrer, 1966; Suzuki et al., 1972; Wong-Riley, 1972; Barron et al., 1973; Fox, 1973). In the present study some cells displayed features which might be indicative of cell degeneration (Fig. 35). In the following section data will be discussed which indicates that the myelin-covered microglial cells do in fact to a large extent undergo degeneration.

In many of the myelin-covered microglial cells smooth intracytoplasmic membranes were found (Figs. 22a and c). Tehse may be related to an autophagocytic process. They seemed to originate from tubules and vesicles probably belonging to the Golgi apparatus or smooth endoplasmic reticulum (Fig. 22c). Membranes limiting the autophagosomes have in many situations been shown to originate from these cell organelles (Ericsson et al., 1965; Glinsmann and Ericsson, 1966; Fedorko et al., 1968; Arstila and Trump, 1968). Similar membranes seem to have been observed in macrophages during direct Wallerian degeneration in the spinal cord and thalamus of cats (Bignami and Ralston, 1969).

To sum up, the myelin-covered microglial cells seem to be characterized by 1. an appearance early in the degenerative process 2. a complete covering of myelin 3. a structure similar to microglial cells found in the control material 4. the occurrence of intracytoplasmic membrane-bounded bodies, which may reflect a participation in the phagocytosis primarily of degenerating axoplasm but also of degenerating myelin. 5. the occurrence of intracytoplasmic membrane-bounded bodies and sometimes smooth membranes both of which might reflect an autophagocytic process terminating in degeneration of the glial cell.

Myelin-covered glial cells have been described during direct Wallerian degeneration, too. In a light microscopical study on the rabbit, monkey and human spinal cord Jakob (1913) described myelin-covered glial cells which he termed "myeloclasts". Similar findings were later made in the rabbit spinal cord (Spatz, 1921; Cramer and Alpers, 1932) and the baboon spinal cord (Daniel and Strich, 1969). Myelin-covered glial cells have also been found during electron microscopical studies of direct Wallerian degeneration, in the avian optic nerve (Gray and Hamlyn, 1962) in the lateral vestibular nucleus (Mugnaini et al., 1967), in the spinal cord and thalamus of the cat (Bignami and Ralston, 1969) and in the kitten spinal cord (Hildebrand, 1971 b). In this context the demonstration of astrocytic processes within myelin sheaths of rat optic nerve fibres following eye enucleation (McMahan, 1967) should also be mentioned.

In view of the large number of ultrastructural studies made on direct Wallerian degeneration it is surprising that myelin-covered glial cells have so seldom been reported. Two facts may be relevant in this context. Firstly, most ultrastructural studies on direct Wallerian degeneration in fibre tracts have been made on rats. Secondly, most ultrastructural studies on other species than the rat have dealt with the degeneration of terminal fibres and axon terminals. It is therefore possible that species differences and regional differences in the glial reaction to degenerative changes in different parts of the degenerating nerve fibre may account for the few reports on myelin-covered glial cells during direct Wallerian degeneration.

It is tempting to suggest that the "myeloclasts" of Jakob (1913) correspond to the myelin-covered microglial cells observed in the present study. "Myeloclasts" appeared early during the process of degeneration, they seemed to be completely enclosed by myelin and they degenerated. They also appeared to take part in the break-down of degenerating myelinated nerve fibres, although this activity was considered to be directed against myelin and not primarily against axoplasm, as the present study indicates for the myelin-covered microglial cells. Based on observations from material where silver impregnation methods were used to demonstrate glial cells, Cramer and Alpers (1932) arrived at the conclusion that the "myeloclasts" were derived from oligodendrocytes. Bignami and Ralston (1969) seem to accept this conclusion as being applicable to the cells they observed during direct Wallerian degeneration in the spinal cord and thalamus of the cat. From their study it is not clear whether the glial cells were completely surrounded by myelin, or whether they contained membrane-bounded bodies of the type observed here. It is obvious, however, that their cells did not show the other structural characteristics of the myelin-covered microglial cells observed here.

If the observations by Bignami and Ralston (1969) are representative of the ultrastructural appearance of the early stages of direct Wallerian degeneration in the cat, the following questions arise: 1. Are the myelin-covered microglial cells characteristic for indirect Wallerian degeneration in the kitten ? 2. Are they characteristic for indirect Wallerian in both immature and mature animals ? 3. Are they characteristic for Wallerian degeneration, both direct and indirect, in the kitten ?

That myelin-covered microglial cells occur during direct Wallerian degeneration in the kitten is indicated by the study of Hildebrand (1971 b). The structural details of these cells and their relation to the process of direct Wallerian degeneration remain to be demonstrated, however.

Nature of the Degenerating Glial Cells

A significant increase in the number of degenerating glial cells occurred on the operated side. That these cells were actually in a state of degeneration was indicated by the pyknotic nucleus (or part of the nucleus) and by the disorganisation of the intracytoplasmic membrane systems. The circumstance leading to the increased number of these cells is considered to be the degeneration of at least a majority of the myelin-covered microglial cells. Firstly, the degenerating glial cells like the myelin-covered microglial cells often had a myelin covering (Figs. 36, 37) and in some instances were completely enveloped by myelin. Secondly, the degenerating glial cells appeared at a time when myelin-covered microglial cells became less frequent (cf. Diagram 1). Furthermore lamellated bodies (cf. Fig. 36) and lipid droplets were often observed in both degenerating glial cells and in myelin-covered microglial cells.

In the cytoplasm of many myelin-covered microglial cells autophagosome-like structures were found (Figs. 31, 32 and 33). In a few cases such cells appeared to be at an early stage of cell degeneration (Fig. 35). It seems reasonable therefore, to assume that the occurrence of presumed autophagosomes in myelin-covered microglial cells is an early event in a process terminating in degeneration of the glial cell as demonstrated above. Whether all myelin-covered microglial cells degenerate cannot be decided from the present study, but the number of degenerating glial cells seemed consistent with complete or almost complete elimination of the former.

Degenerating glial cells have been described under several different experimental and pathological conditions. Light microscopically, glial cells with a pyknotic nucleus have been noted in conjunction with transneuronal degeneration in the pontine nuclei of kittens (Torvik, 1956; Trumpy, 1971). Electron microscopically, degenerating glial cells have been described under some demyelinating conditions (Lampert, 1967 b; Howell and Kidd, 1969; Suzuki et al., 1969; Raine and Bornstein, 1970), in immature rats treated with the hypercholesteremic drug AY 9944 (Suzuki et al., 1971), in the jimpy mouse (Privat et al., 1972), in cuprizone-intoxicated mice (Blakemore, 1972 b) and in the subependymal plate of INH-treated dogs (Blakemore et al., 1972). Such cells also occur infrequently in the brains of normal adult animals (Pannese and Ferrannini, 1967; Mori and Leblond, 1969 b) and more frequently during the normal postnatal development of large myelinated fibres in the spinal cord (Spatz, 1918; Hildebrand, 1971 b).

Of particular relevance to the present findings are reports on degenerating glial cells during direct Wallerian degeneration. In his study on direct Wallerian degeneration in the rabbit, monkey and human spinal cord, Jakob (1913) described how the "myeloclasts" (cf. above) rapidly developed nuclear pyknosis and karyorrhexis, i.e. degenerated. These findings have been confirmed in other light microscopical studies (Spatz, 1921; Daniel and Strich, 1969). In an electron microscopical study on direct Wallerian degeneration in the cat spinal cord and thalamus "round cell nuclei with very scant cytoplasm or no cytoplasm at all were found surrounded by degenerated myelin sheaths" (Bignami and Ralston, 1969). These cells were considered to be the counterpart of Jakob's myeloclasts. Degenerating glial cells which were often covered by myelin have been described in the kitten spinal cord after dorsal root transections (Hildebrand, 1971 b). As a whole, however, there are few reports on degenerating glial cells during direct Wallerian degeneration. A similar statement has already been made in relation to the myelin-covered microglial cells (see above). Here too, species differences and regional differences in the glial reaction to degenerating changes in different parts of the degenerating nerve fibre may account for the discrepancy between the vast number of studies on direct Wallerian degeneration and the few reports on degenerating glial cells during that process. The reason why glial cells degenerate during direct Wallerian degeneration and during the indirect Wallerian degeneration studied here, is unknown. Spatz (1921) considered the degeneration of the "myeloclasts" as "Opfertod". Daniel and Strich (1969) suggested that these cells "literally suffocated" within the closed bag of myelin. At least it seems reasonable to assume that the transport of essential nutrients to the myelin-covered glial cells is delayed by the compact myelin covering.

Some of the degenerating glial cells seen by various authors in light and electron microscopical studies of direct Wallerian degeneration probably correspond to those described in the present study. At the same time it seems correct to state that our knowledge of the structural details of degenerating glial cells and their relation to the process of fibre degeneration during direct Wallerian degeneration in adult and immature animals is poor. It also remains to be shown whether such cells occur during indirect Wallerian degeneration in adult animals.

The Late Reaction of Microglial Cells

Microglial cells situated outside myelin were found to phagocytose degenerating structures (Figs. 38, 39 and 40). In addition to their different position in relation to myelin, these glial cells differed from the myelin-covered microglial cells in three principal respects: 1. Microglial cells outside myelin appeared later during the process of degeneration (cf. Diagram 1) 2. The activity of the cells seemed to be directed primarily towards degenerating myelin. 3. No evidence for degeneration of these cells was found.

It seems likely that these microglial cells correspond to the phagocytic cells described previously in several studies on direct Wallerian degeneration, such as the "myelophage" in the spinal cord of rabbits and monkeys (Jakob, 1913), the multipotential glial cell in the optic nerve of the rat (Vaughn et al., 1970 and the macrophage in the spinal cord and thalamus of the cat (Bignami and Ralston, 1969). It should be pointed out, however, that the crystalline-like inclusions described in the phagocytes in the two latter studies were rarely observed in the present study. This may be due to differences in the preparatory procedure, to maturational differences or to differences in the process of myelin degeneration.

The classification of the phagocytic cells described here as microglial cells is based purely on structural similarities to microglial cells observed in control material. In many instances of central nervous degeneration, perivascular and/or hematogeneous cells enter the central nervous tissue and become transformed into phagocytes of similar appearance as microglial cells (Russel, 1962; Konigsmark and Sidman, 1963; Blakemore, 1972a; Kitamura et al., 1972; Matthews and Kruger, 1973; Oemichen et al., 1973). Studies with labelling techniques indicate that the phagocytes during direct Wallerian degeneration in the rat optic nerve and in the newborn rabbit spinal cord, are of endogenous origin (Skoff and Vaughn, 1971; Stenwig, 1973). Two findings made in the present study may be relevant in this context, however. Firstly, mitotic cells were observed most frequently between 1 and 2 weeks postoperatively, i.e. shortly before microglial cells outside myelin were most commonly seen. Secondly, two mitotic cells had obviously phagocytosed fragments of degenerating myelinated nerve fibres (Fig. 42). These two findings seem compatible with an endogenous origin for the phagocytic microglial cells located outside myelin.

In summary, the late reaction of microglial cells seems to be essentially similar to the microglial reaction observed during direct Wallerian degeneration in adult animals. Whether this statement is true also for direct Wallerian degeneration in immature animals is not known.

The Reaction of Pericytes

Late during the process of degeneration some pericytes loaded with dense bodies and vacuoles were observed (Fig. 40). Both dense bodies and vacuoles may be sites of lysosomal enzyme activity. In some previous studies on direct Wallerian degeneration, perivascular cells have been allotted a prominent role in the phagocytosis of degenerating structures (Vaughn, 1965; Berger, 1971). Pictures have been presented, too, supposedly showing perivascular cells penetrating the basement membrane to enter the central nervous tissue, possibly to phagocytose degenerating material (see e.g. Bignami and Ralston, 1969). In other studies on direct Wallerian degeneration the perivascular cells are said to undergo little change (Vaughn and Pease, 1970). The findings made here seem to be compatible with the interpretation that degenerating material is transferred to some pericytes for degradation and perhaps excreted into the vascular system. It cannot be excluded, however, that phagocytic cells have moved with their phagocytosed content to a perivascular position, where break-down of the phagocytosed material is completed.

In summary, the comparison of the present findings on indirect Wallerian degeneration with previous findings on direct Wallerian degeneration in adult animals is somewhat hampered by the divergent reports concerning the role of perivascular cells indirect Wallerian degeneration in adult animals. With regard to that process in immature animals nothing seems to be known.

The Formation of a Glial Scar

In the present study it was found that when signs of degeneration became less marked, hypertrophy of astrocytes and proliferation of astrocytic processes became evident (Figs. 44, 45). Astrocytes and their processes seemed to replace degenerated myelinated nerve fibres completely. An astrocytic reaction is also a well known consequence of a great number of experimental and pathological conditions, e.g. traumatic degeneration in the central nervous system (Cajal, 1928b; Rand, 1952; Cavanagh, 1970), radiation lesions (Miquel and Haymaker, 1965; Brownson et al., 1972) and brain edema (Friede, 1965; Hirano, 1969). In such conditions a significant accumulation of glycogen occures in the astrocytes (Shimizu and Hamuro, 1958; Miquel and Haymaker, 1965; Guth and Watson, 1968; Hirano, 1969). This was not the case in the present situation nor in association with direct Wallerian degeneration in adult animals (cf. Bignami and Ralston, 1969; Dunkerley and Duncan, 1969; Vaughn and Pease, 1970; Mossakowski and Penar, 1972).

In immature animals in contrast to adult animals there is not any marked astrocytic reaction to traumatic degeneration (Spatz, 1921; Sumi and Hager, 1968). Studies with aluminium hydroxide injections in young and adult animals indicate that injury to myelinated nerve fibres elicits anastrocytic reaction in contrast to injury of unmyelinated nerve fibres (Fleischauer and Schmalbach, 1968). The prominent astrocytic reaction described here may therefore be related to the considerable degree of myelination of the degenerating nerve fibres. Whether a similar glial reaction occurs also in direct Wallerian degeneration of myelinated nerve fibres in immature animals does not seem to be known.

Possible Signs of Regenerative Activity

Two observations were made which were suggestive of regenerative activity.

1. In some cases axons were seen (Fig. 18) which resembled the proximal stumps of transected regenerating axons in the central (Lampert and Cressman, 1964; Lampert, 1967a) and peripheral nervous systems (Morris et al., 1972). The axons observed here (Fig. 18) may belong to cell bodies which did not undergo retrograde cell *degeneration*. That such cells exist under the present experimental conditions is known from previous studies where roughly one quarter of the hypoglossal neurones in kittens operated on at 5 days of age were shown to survive nerve transection (Grant and Aldskogius, unpublished observations). An alternative explanation is that the axons observed here represent a variety of axonal degeneration. This is supported by the occasional finding of a microglial cell surrounding part of such an axon.

2. Late in the process of degeneration a few oligodendrocytes were found to be surrounded by a couple of myelin lamellae (Fig. 43). Similar findings have been described in direct Wallerian degeneration in rat optic nerve where it has been interpreted as a sign of aberrant remyelination (Vaughn and Pease, 1970), an interpretation which seems reasonable in relation to the present findings, too. The same interpretation has also been offered for the probably related finding of myelinated astrocytic processes late during direct Wallerian degeneration in the cat spinal cord and thalamus (Bignami and Ralston, 1968, 1969).

Indications Concerning the Appearance of Indirect Wallerian Degeneration in Adult Animals

In the present study observations on indirect Wallerian degeneration were made on a group of kittens 2–28 days old at operation (cf. Table 1). Although the number of degenerating structures was considerably less in kittens operated on at 21–28 days than in those of a lower age at operation, the fundamental qualitative changes were the same. This may indicate that the appearance of indirect Wallerian degeneration in adult cats is similar to the description given here.

Light microscopical studies with silver impregnation methods indicate that indirect Wallerian degeneration in the kitten has a characteristic granular appearance (Grant and Aldskogius, 1967; Grant, 1968; Grant and Westman, 1969), as opposed to the fragmented fibre appearance of direct Wallerian degeneration in adult animals. It seems clear from the few published descriptions and pictures of indirect Wallerian degeneration in silver impregnated sections from adult animals, that thalamo-cortical fibres undergoing this type of degeneration show a fragmented fibre appearance (Powell and Cowan, 1964; Guillery, 1967; Wong-Riley, 1972). In these studies, however, the cell bodies giving rise to the degenerating fibres were not only deefferented, but were also in part deafferented by the lesions which caused the degeneration of the cell bodies. Therefore, the indirect Wallerian degeneration described in these studies is not fully comparable to that in the kitten studies mentioned above, where the degenerating cell bodies have been purely deefferented. The latter holds true for the retrograde cell degeneration causing the fibre degeneration described in the isthmo-optic tract and the trochlear nerve of adult pigeons (Cowan *et al.*, 1961). Unfortunately, it is not possible to draw safe conclusions from the data presented in that study about the appearance of the indirect Wallerian degeneration in these two systems.

The Dynamic Picture of Indirect Wallerian Degeneration in the Kitten—A Working Hypothesis

On the basis of the observations made in the present study, a tentative interpretation is presented of the dynamic events occurring during indirect Wallerian degeneration in the kitten. A study based on static pictures showing only the morphological aspects of a dynamic process can at most give only indications of the functional changes. An attempt to synthesize these static pictures into a dynamic process may help to emphasize, however, the fundamental problems which require further studies.

As a result of the break-down of metabolism in the parent cell bodies degenerative changes occur in their axons. Stimulated by these degenerative changes microglial cells migrate into certain portions of the myelin sheath entering at nodes of Ranvier. The function of these microglial cells is firstly to remove degenerating axoplasm and secondly to remove some of their myelin envelope. Possibly as a result of impairment of nutritional transport through their myelin covering these microglial cells develop foci of cytoplasmic degradation and ultimately disintegrate and die. The covering myelin also disintegrates.

Other portions of the myelinated nerve fibres (or other nerve fibres) undergo a different series of changes. The degenerating axoplasm shrinks and causes secondary changes in the surrounding myelin leading to the appearance of myelin bodies. This process of myelin sheath disintegration stimulates the arrival of another set of microglial cells. The myelin bodies are phagocytosed by these cells and further degradated.

Simultaneously with the removal of the degenerating structures, the missing nerve fibres are replaced by hypertrophied astrocytes and their processes.

Several problems have to be solved before this hypothetical picture could be accepted. It is necessary, for instance, to prove that the present interpretation of the membrane-bounded structures in the myelin-covered microglial cells is correct. It is also necessary to establish how these cells come to be covered by myelin and what is the mechanism of their degeneration. If the hypothesis outlined above was shown to be valid then one must ask why degenerating axoplasm seems to follow two different courses in its degeneration.

The Ultrastructural Basis of the Nauta Picture of Indirect Wallerian Degeneration

In Nauta impregnated sections from the kitten, indirect Wallerian degeneration appears mainly as collections of impregnated granules. Direct Wallerian degeneration in adult animals has, on the other hand a typical fragmented fibre appearance.

There is general agreement that electron-dense axons are impregnated with suppressive silver methods (Eager and Barrnett, 1966; Heimer and Ekholm, 1967; Heimer and Peters, 1968; Walberg, 1971, 1972). This is probably the ultrastructural basis for the impregnated fragmented fibres seen during direct Wallerian degeneration in adult animals and for the few impregnated fragmented fibres which are seen during indirect Wallerian degeneration in the kitten.

Whether this is also the ultrastructural basis for the impregnated granules seen in indirect Wallerian degeneration of the kitten cannot be stated at present. Two other possible explanations for these granules might be the impregnation of myelin bodies or parts or myelin bodies and the impregnation of the membrane-bounded bodies in myelin-covered microglial cells. To define the ultrastructural counterpart of the impregnated granules which characterize indirect Wallerian degeneration in the kitten, it is necessary to study silver impregnated sections in the electron microscope. In a later publication, results obtained from such a study will be presented.

Does the Ultrastructural Appearance of Indirect Wallerian Degeneration Differ from that of Direct Wallerian Degeneration?

From the preceding discussion it is evident that the question whether morphological differences exist between indirect and direct Wallerian degeneration cannot be answered at present. Despite the fact that this study has been made on immature animals the findings necessarily had to be discussed largely in the light of previous studies on direct Wallerian degeneration in *adult* animals, due to the fact that our knowledge of the ultrastructural changes during direct Wallerian degeneration in immature animals is so limited. To answer the question raised above, this knowledge must be extended. In the following study an attempt in this direction has been made.

V. Summary

In many parts of the kitten central nervous system a lesion causing damage to a nerve fibre results in degeneration of its cell body. Secondary to this, degeneration occurs in that part of the fibre lying between the parent cell body and the site of lesion. This degeneration has been termed indirect Wallerian fibre degeneration, as opposed to direct Wallerian fibre degeneration, which refers to fibre degeneration distal to the site of lesion. In contrast to the direct Wallerian degeneration, the indirect Wallerian degeneration has not been the subject of any systematic ultrastructural study before. In the present study the ultrastructural characteristics of indirect Wallerian degeneration have been studied in the intramedullary root fibre region of the hypoglossal nerve of 58 kittens subjected to peripheral nerve transection at an age of 2–28 days and surviving for 1–60 days postoperatively.

After a period of 3–6 days (the length depending upon the age of the animals at operation) degenerative changes occur, which first manifest themselves as an increased electron density of axons of myelinated fibres and later as axonal shrinkage and fragmentation. Ultimately collapse of the myelin enwrapping the shrunken axons occurs giving rise to myelin bodies. Simultaneously loops of double-layered myelin appear, sometimes partially enveloping oligodendrocytes.

At an early stage of the degenerative process one finds microglial cells which are completely covered by myelin. These cells appear to primarily participate in the phagocytosis of axoplasm but also to be involved in the disintegration of its myelin covering. Structures suggestive of autophagosomes occur in these myelin-covered microglial cells.

At a later stage a large number of glial cells showing clear signs of degeneration appear. They are often completely covered by myelin. The results indicate that the majority of these degenerating glial cells are derived from the above-mentioned myelin-covered microglial cells.

Within 1 week after the first signs of axonal degeneration, microglial cells located outside myelin sheaths appear in increased numbers. They show signs of phagocytosis of degenerating myelin sheaths, degenerating myelinated nerve fibres and degenerating glial cells. These microglial cells outside myelin sheaths do not seem to undergo degeneration.

Pericytes containing large numbers of dense bodies and vacuoles are found at a late stage of the degenerative process.

Concomitant with the disappearance of the degeneration nerve fibres, hypertrophic astrocytes containing greatly increased numbers of various cell organelles are seen. In addition, a proliferation of astrocytic processes occurs.

Myelin-covered microglial cells of the type described here have not been clearly implicated in the process of Wallerian degeneration before. The possibility that this cell type may be characteristic for indirect Wallerian degeneration in the kitten is discussed.

PART II. DIRECT WALLERIAN DEGENERATION

I. Introduction

In the previous study (Part I) a description was given of the ultrastructural changes occurring during *indirect* Wallerian degeneration in the intramedullary root fibre region of the kitten hypoglossal nerve. One of the striking features of this degeneration process was the appearance at an early stage of microglial cells completely covered by myelin, which apparently participated in phagocytosis of degenerating axoplasm and to a small extent of their own myelin covering. Evidence was obtained indicating that the numerous degenerating glial cells seen somewhat later in the degeneration process were derived from these myelin-covered microglial cells. Since glial cells of the type described in the previous study have never been implicated in the process of *direct* Wallerian degeneration, the possibility exists that they may in fact be characteristic for indirect Wallerian degeneration. However, this possibility cannot be adequately assessed unless our present rather scanty knowledge concerning the early glial reaction during direct Wallerian degeneration is extended. Therefore the present study has been undertaken to examine the ultrastructural changes during direct Wallerian degeneration in the kitten, with particular reference to the possible occurrence of myelin-covered microglial cells and degenerating glial cells of the type described in the previous study (see Part I). Since no systematic ultrastructural study on direct Wallerian degeneration in immature animals seem to exist, observations on changes in the myelinated nerve fibres and the different types of glial cells have been included.

It will be shown that in general the qualitative changes during direct Wallerian degeneration correspond to those described during indirect Wallerian degeneration (see Part I). In particular, similar myelin-covered microglial cells and degenerating glial cells were observed during direct Wallerian degeneration. The results indicated, however, that quantitative differences with regard to the occurrence of these cells might exist between the two types of Wallerian degeneration.

II. Material and Methods

5 kittens aged 5 to 17 days at operation and with postoperative survival times of 6 hours to 23 days were used for this study (Table 3).

Before the operation anaesthesia was induced by intraperitoneal injection of Mebumal® (30 mg/kg). This was sometimes supplemented by 0.5–1.0 ml of 0.5% Xylocain-Exadrin® (Astra, Södertälje, Sweden) administered locally. The dorsal surfaces of the occipital bone and atlas were then exposed by a midline incision through the skin and muscles. The posterior atlanto-occipital membrane was cut open and part of the occipital bone removed. The dura and arachnoid membranes covering the dorsal aspects of the cerebellum and brain stem were cut open. After careful dissection the posterior part of the cerebellum was gently lifted to expose the caudal part of the rhomboid fossa. Using a fine needle, a unilateral, rostro-caudal

Table 3. Summary of time data and extent of lesions for the animals used in the study

Age at operation (days)	Survival time	Part of the hypoglossal nucleus affected by lesion
14	6 hours	rostral 1/2
17	20 hours	rostral 1/3
6	2 days	rostral 1/3
15	2 days	rostral 1/3
6	3 days	rostral 1/3
8	3 days	middle 1/3
11	3 days	rostral 1/2
5	4 days	middle 1/3
6	5 days	rostral 1/3
8	6 days	middle 1/3
7	7 days	rostral 1/3
5	8 days	rostral 1/3
8	10 days	middle 1/3
14	10 days	rostral 1/2
17	23 days	rostral tip

lesion of the hypoglossal nucleus was made mechanically. Minimal bleeding occurred during this procedure. The muscles and skin were sutured. Immediately after the operation the animals were given penicillin intramuscularly in the gluteal region. They seemed to be in good condition during the whole postoperative period.

The animals were sacrificed by perfusion. Under Mebumal® anaesthesia the chest was opened and a cannula inserted into the ascending aorta. A rinsing solution (pH 7.35–7.45, temp. 38° C) consisting of a 300 mOsm Millonigbuffer (1961) with 2.7% Dextran T 40 (Pharmacia, Uppsala, Sweden) was perfused for about 30 secs. at a pressure of 100–120 mm Hg. A warm (38°C) fixative solution was then perfused at the same pressure for 3–4 min after which it was gradually replaced by a cold (7°C) fixative solution perfused at a pressure of 70–90 mm Hg. The fixative solution consisted of 5% glutaraldehyde in a 300 mOsm Millonig buffer (1961) with 2.7% Dextran T 40. The pH was 7.35–7.45 and the total tonicity 800–850 mOsm/l.

After perfusion the tissue was treated as described in the previous study (see Part I). During the dissection of the intramedullary root fibre region of the hypoglossal nerve, care was taken not to include the region close to the ventral edge of the lesion or the region immediately beneath the ventral surface of the medulla.

1 μm thick sections cut from each of the small blocks prepared from the root fibre region (cf. Part I) were examined in the light microscope after staining with toluidine-blue. Small blocks from the non-operated side were mainly used for light microscopy. Small blocks from the operated side were prepared for electron microscopy as described in the previous study (see Part I). Short series (20–30 sections) of ultrathin sections were cut from each block. Additional longer series (300–400 sections) were cut from some blocks. The sections were examined in a Philips 300 EM electron microscope.

The medullary slices which contained the lesions and from which the small blocks were cut (cf. Fig. 46) were dehydrated in a graded series of alcohol, embedded in paraffin and cut in serial transverse sections at 20 μm. Every second section was stained with cresyl violet and every second according to van Gieson. Examination in the light microscope enabled the extent of the lesions to be entered on schematic drawings prepared from a series of thionin-stained sections of the medulla of a 10 day old kitten.

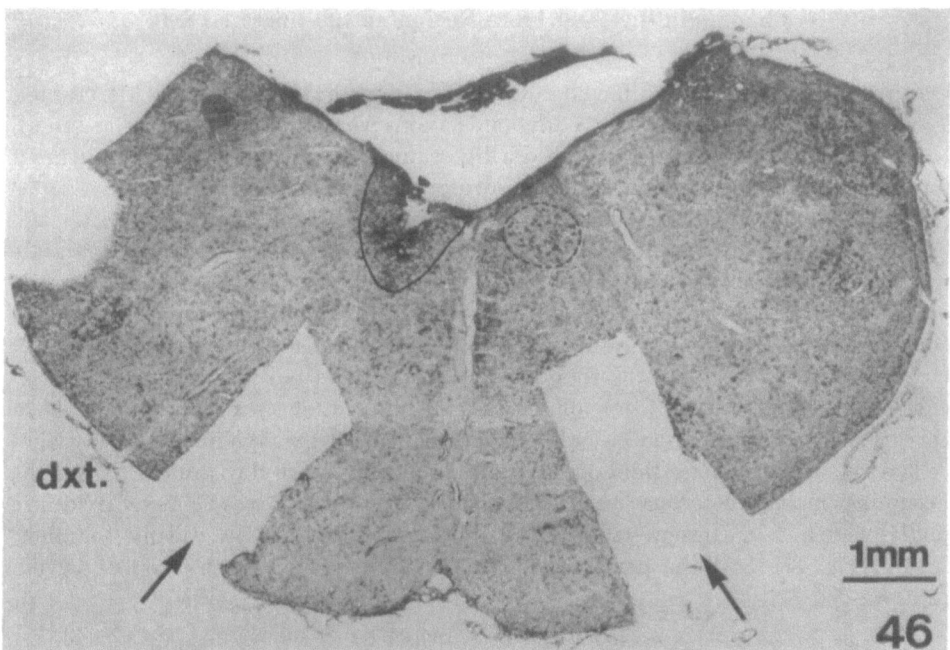

Fig. 46. 15 days at operation, 2 days survival. Transverse, Nissl stained section of the medulla oblongata. Solid line indicates border of the lesion. Dashed line indicates border of the contralateral (normal) hypoglossal nucleus. Part of the medulla containing the intramedullary root fibre region of the hypoglossal nerve at this level has been cut out (arrow) for embedding in Epon. It should be noted that the root region just beneath the ventral surface in the medulla was not processed for electron microscopy

III. Observations

A. Methods

Uniformly satisfactory preservation was not obtained in every animal. In all animals, however, several blocks of the intramedullary root fibre region of the hypoglossal nerve showed satisfactory preservation. The quality of the preservation seemed to be generally lower than in a previous study in which a peripheral rather than a central lesion was made (see Part I).

B. Lesions

In all animals the lesion affected the hypoglossal nucleus or the intramedullary root fibres of the hypoglossal nerve only on one side. In 5 kittens the lesions affected the rostral half of the hypoglossal nucleus, in 7 the rostral third, in 4 the middle third and in one only the rostral tip (Table 3). This last had the longest survival time (23 days). In most animals the majority of hypoglossal neurones at the level of the lesions seemed to have been destroyed (Fig. 46) and in animals with postoperative survival times of 2 days or more the remainder often displayed chromatolytic changes. The lesions regularly included areas outside the hypoglossal nucleus (cf. Fig. 46).

C. Changes in the Root Fibre Region on the Operated Side
a) Light Microscopy

In the animal surviving for 20 hours after the operation, a few darkly stained axons were observed. From 2 to 5 days such axons were numerous (Fig. 47a and c). From 2 to 23 days postoperatively darkly stained, round or irregularly outlined formations were seen, sometimes showing alternating dark and light zones (Fig. 47b, c and d). These formations were numerous from 3 to 10 days after the operation. Glial cells enveloped by myelin were observed from 2 to 10 days after the operation. Some of these cells had a heterochromatic nucleus (Fig. 47a), while others had an euchromatic nucleus (Fig. 47d). The former type was particularly common at the 2 day stage and not seen at all from the 6th postoperative day onwards. The latter type was found from 3 to 10 days but was in no case particularly common. Examination of serial semithin sections through some cells of this type revealed them to be only partially enclosed by myelin. At 6 days glial cells with a dark nucleus, lipid droplets and inclusions started to appear (Fig. 47f), becoming more numerous until the 10th day. From 2 to 23 days pyknotic bodies were found. These were surrounded by a vacuolated or practically "empty" region (Fig. 47e). At the periphery of these regions myelin was often observed.

b) Electron Microscopy
α) Changes in Axons and Myelin Sheaths

Changes on the operated side were present as early as 6 hours after the operation. In some axons filaments were more closely packed than normally and occupied the central part of the axon, while vesicular profiles, lamellated structures and mitochondria (sometimes of an unusual appearance) were located in the periphery (Fig. 48). Such axons were occasionally still seen 20 hours after operation. At that stage a few axons with very tightly packed filaments and microtubules were also encountered (Fig. 49).

The darkly stained axons seen in the light microscope corresponded to axons with an electron-dense matrix and deranged mitochondria. Such axons, seen on some occasions as early as 20 hours after the operation, were numerous and dominated the field of degeneration at 2 days (Fig. 50). They were frequent between 2 and 5 days postoperatively and continued to be found until 10 days. In these axons no filaments or tubules could be identified and the mitochondria were round, often swollen and without visible cristae (Fig. 50). The amount of glial cytoplasm beneath the innermost layer of the enwrapping myelin sheath often was increased (Figs. 50, 51). Nerve fibres showing obvious shrinkage of their axoplasm were seen occasionally at 2 days but were numerous from 3 to 10 days (Fig. 51).

The most prominent sign of myelin sheath degeneration was the presence of myelin bodies, i.e. layers of myelin irregularly wrinkled and sometimes folded upon each other (Figs. 50, 51). These myelin bodies were the counterpart of the darkly stained, round or irregular formations seen in the light microscope (cf Fig. 47b, c and d). Between the myelin layers was a region which could be "empty" (Fig. 50) or filled with cytoplasmic-like material (Figs. 50, 51). Myelin bodies were observed from 2 to 23 days, being most frequent in the 3 to 10 day

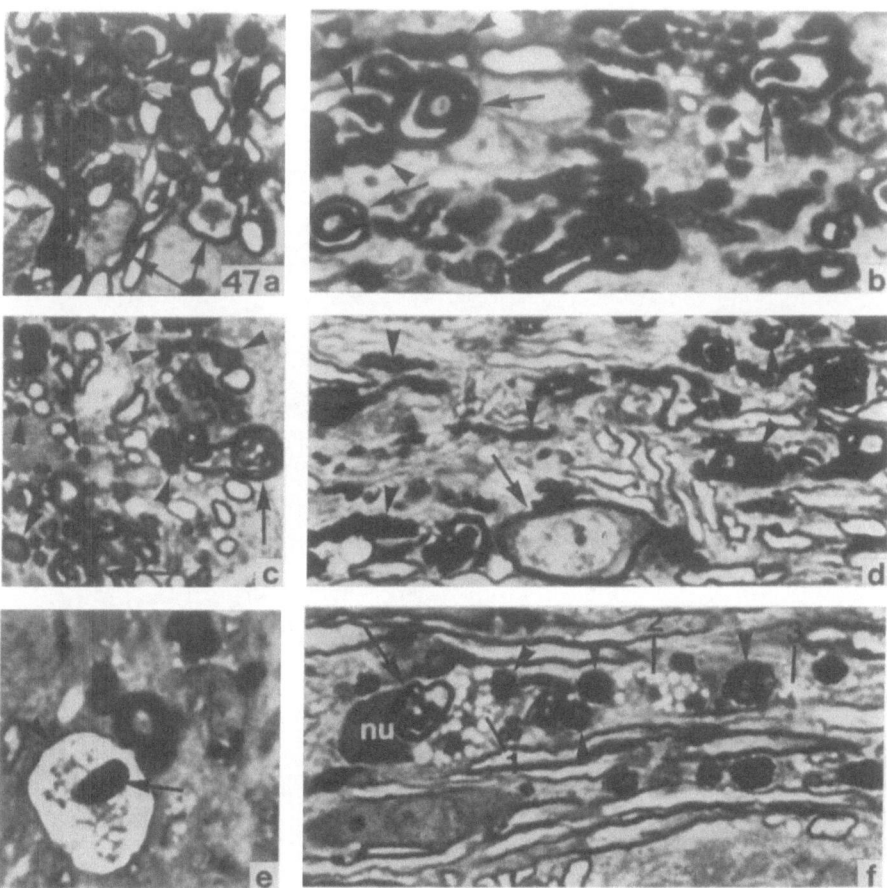

Fig. 47 a—f. Light micrographs of 1 μm thick, toluidine-blue stained sections from the intra-medullary root fibres of the hypoglossal nerve. × 1650. a 15 days at operation, 2 days survival. Transverse section. Several darkly stained axons are seen (arrowheads). In addition two glial cells (one of which with a heterochromatic nucleus) surrounded by myelin can be seen (arrows). b 11 days at operation, 3 days survival. Longitudinal section. Several darkly stained axons are seen (arrowheads). In addition a few formations (arrows) having a slightly irregular outline and showing alternating light areas and dark layers of myelin. c 8 days at operation, 3 days survival. Transverse section. A great number of darkly stained axons (arrowheads) and a few irregularly outlined formations (arrows) which seem to consist of myelin layers interposed with light areas. d 7 days at operation, 7 days survival. Longitudinal section. Several fragments of degenerating fibres are seen (arrowheads). In addition a glial cell, (arrow) with an euchromatic nucleus, is seen to be surrounded by myelin. e 14 days at operation, 10 days survival. Transverse section. A pyknotic body (arrow) is surrounded by a reticular structure which in turn is surrounded by an "empty" space. A thin dark line, possibly remnants of myelin, is seen (arrowhead). Above, three fragments of degenerating fibres. f 8 days at operation, 10 days survival. Longitudinal section. To the left a dark glial cell (nucleus = nu), probably belonging to a large, myelin-like inclusion (arrow) and several lipid droplets (1). A great number of other structures which may be inclusions in the same or in another glial cell are seen (arrowheads) as well as two groups of lipid droplets (2 and 3)

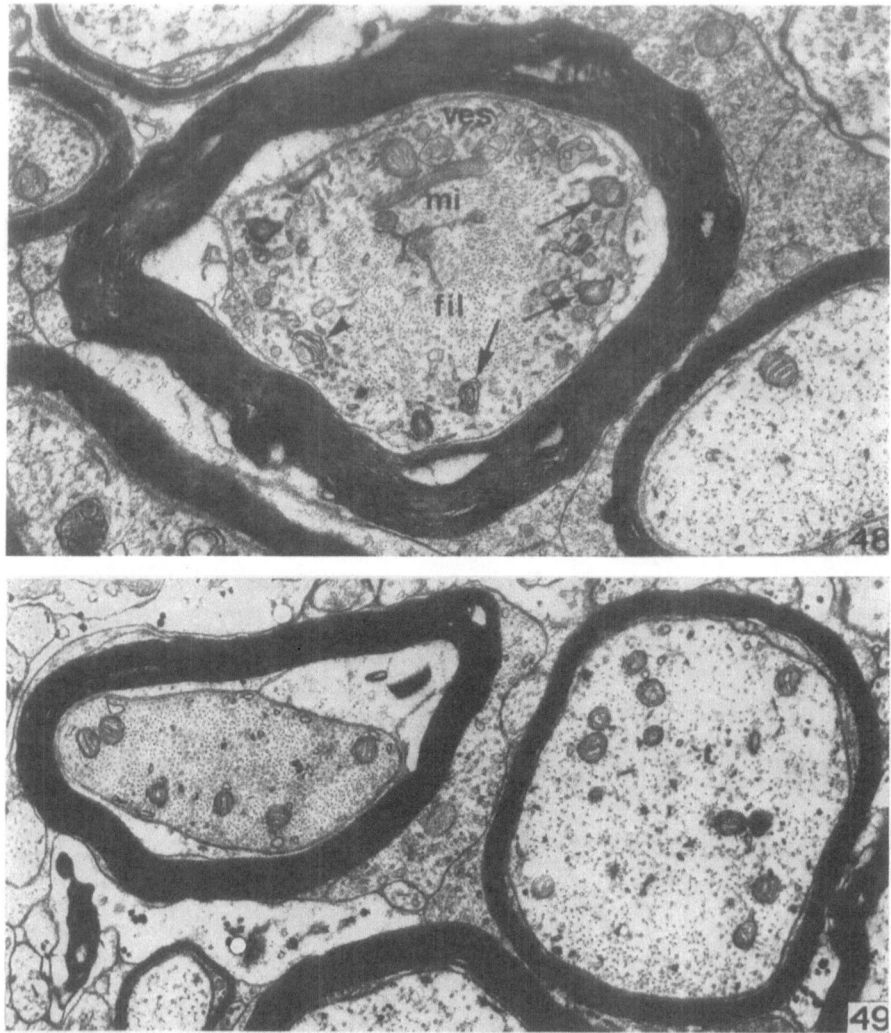

Fig. 48. 14 days at operation, 6 hours survival. Transverse section. A myelinated axon having closely packed filaments (*fil*) centrally and various forms of structures peripherally, such as vesicles (*ves*), lamellar bodies (arrows) and mitochondria (*mi*). In one of these (arrowhead) the cristae are of unusually high electron density. Note the thick myelin sheath. × 27500

Fig. 49. 17 days at operation, 20 hours survival. Transverse section. At left a myelinated axon with closely arranged filaments and tubules. The mitochondria appear normal. At right a normal-looking myelinated axons. × 18000

Fig. 50. 15 days at operation, 2 days survival. Transverse section. Several myelinated, electron-dense axons. Filaments and tubules are not visible in the electron-dense matrix. Mitochondria in some of the electron-dense fibres appear enlarged (*mi*). At some places there is a rather thick layer of glial cytoplasm surrounding the electron-dense axon (arrows). Note myelin body (*my*) formed out of four concentrically arranged layers of myelin. A thin rim of cytoplasm resembling glial cytoplasm (*gl*) is seen between the two outermost myelin layers. × 14200

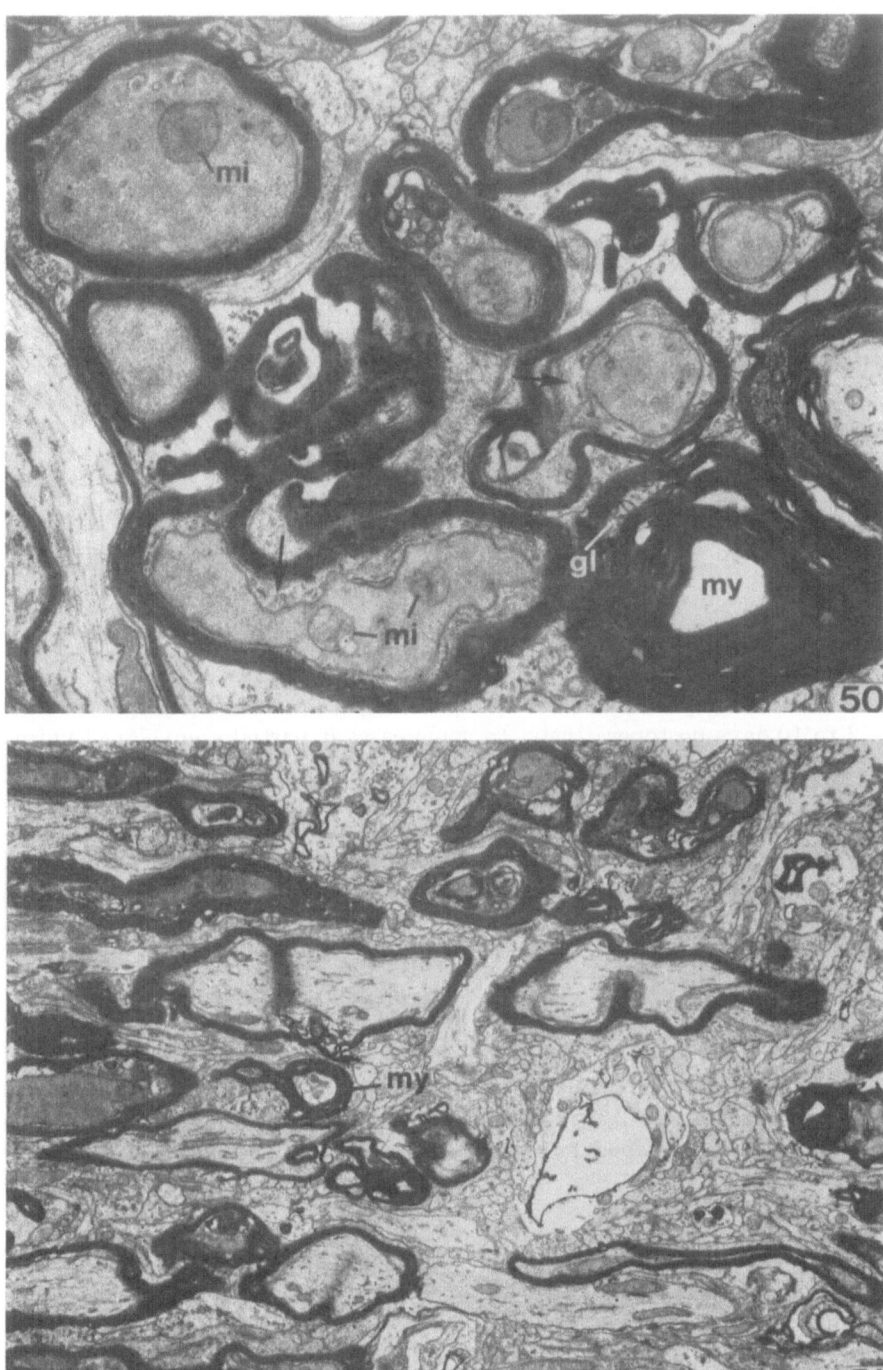

Fig. 51. 8 days at operation, 3 days survival. Longitudinal section. Several myelinated, electron-dense somewhat shrunken axons are seen. In addition there is a myelin body (*my*), which contains a centrally located shrunken cytoplasmic-like structure. × 5600

lesions of the hypoglossal nucleus. Areas with hatched lines indicate the time periods when the changes which were observed in myelinated nerve fibres and glial cells following ipsilateral lesions of the hypoglossal nucleus. Areas with hatched lines indicate the time periods when the different changes were most frequently observed

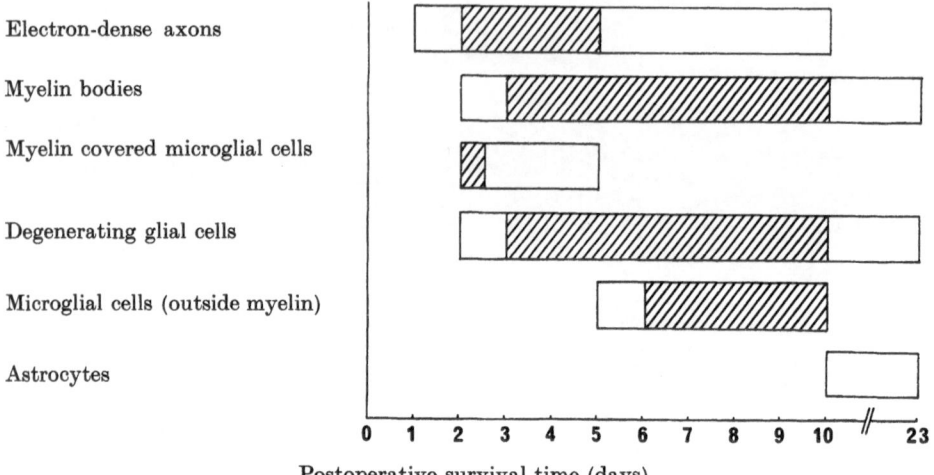

Postoperative survival time (days)

period. Aberrant myelin, i.e. double layers of myelin forming loops were seen from 2 to 10 days postoperatively. In some cases it partially enveloped normal-looking oligodendrocytes (Fig. 52).

Largely related to the variation in size of the lesions of the hypoglossal nucleus in different animals, differences were found in the total number of degenerating fibres in animals with the same postoperative survival time. It was evident, however, that in all cases with survival times of 2 to 10 days, the number of degenerating fibres clearly exceeded the maximum number ever seen in cases of indirect Wallerian degeneration of the kitten hypoglossal nerve described in the earlier study (see Part I).

β) Changes in Glial Cells (cf. Diagram 2)

From 2 to 5 days after the operation glial cells resembling microglial cells in the normal intramedullary root fibre region of the kitten hypoglossal nerve were found to be enveloped by a single layer of normal-looking myelin. These

Fig. 52. 5 days at operation, 4 days survival. Longitudinal section. Oligodendrocyte partially surrounded by aberrant myelin. Note the close contact between the two myelin layers except where they are in continuity (arrows). × 8500

Fig. 53. 15 days at operation, 2 days survival. Transverse section. Myelin-covered microglial cell. Note clumping of chromatin in nucleus (*nu*). In the cytoplasm, which is moderately electron-dense there are scattered ribosomes, vesicular profiles (*ves*), a few short membranes of rough-surfaced endoplasmic reticulum (*er*) and one mitochondrion (*mi*). Note glial processes (*gp*) invaginating the perikaryal cytoplasm. Below, a degenerating axon surrounded, and also penetrated (arrowheads) by glial cytoplasm. × 15000

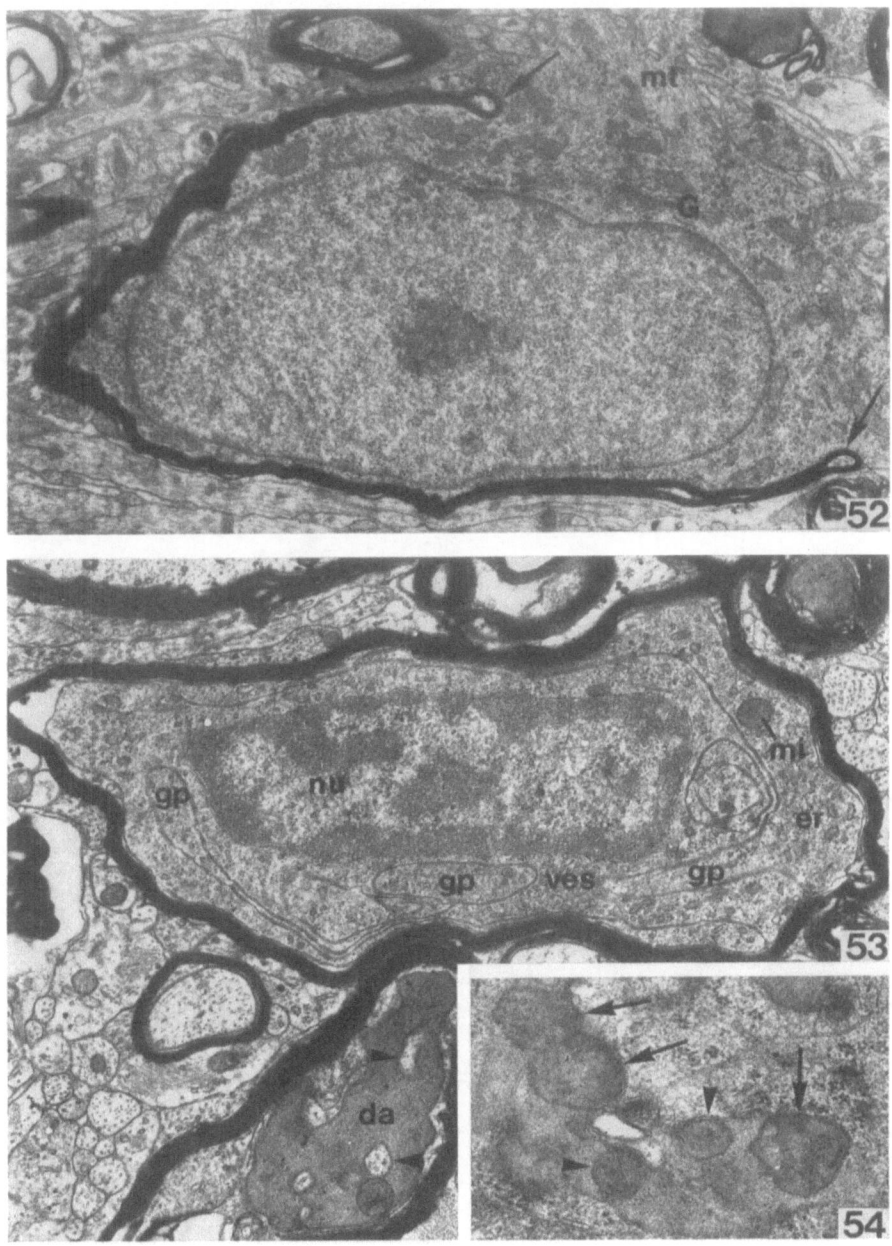

Fig. 54. 15 days at operation, 2 days survival. Longitudinal section. Membrane-bounded body in myelin-covered microglial cell. The body has an irregular outline, and a dense matrix in which three large (arrows) and two small (arrowheads) mitochondria-like formations are found.
× 27000

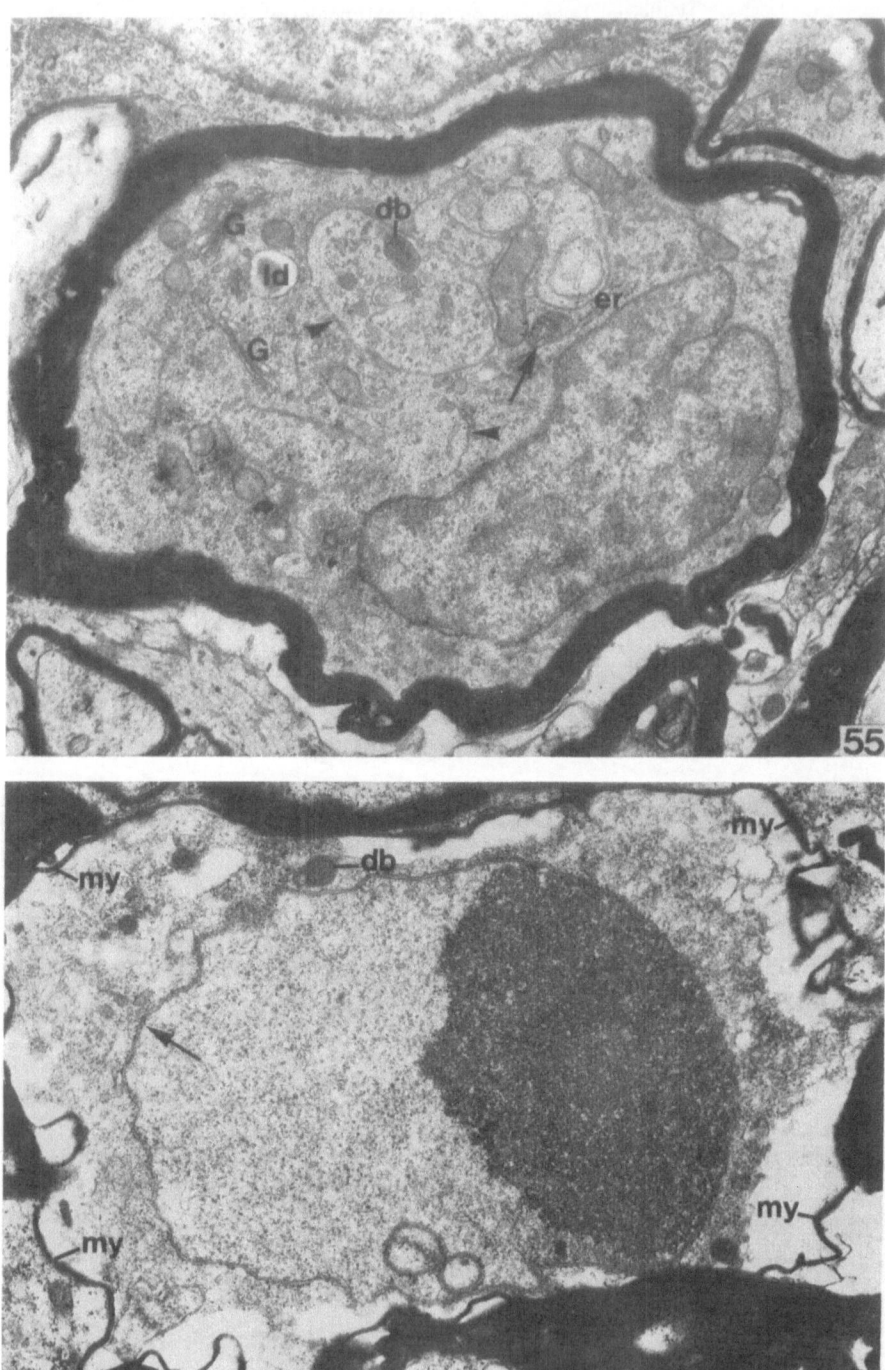

Fig. 55. 15 days at operation, 2 days survival. Transverse section. Myelin-covered microglial cell. The nucleus shows moderate clumping of chromatin. The cytoplasm is abundant and contains scattered ribosomes, Golgi apparatus (*G*) with some narrow cisterns, a few short rows of rough-surfaced endoplasmic reticulum (*er*), one lipid droplet (*ld*), one dense body (*db*), one multivesicular body (arrow), and a few intracellular membranes (arrowhead). Note normal-looking myelin around the cell. × 14700

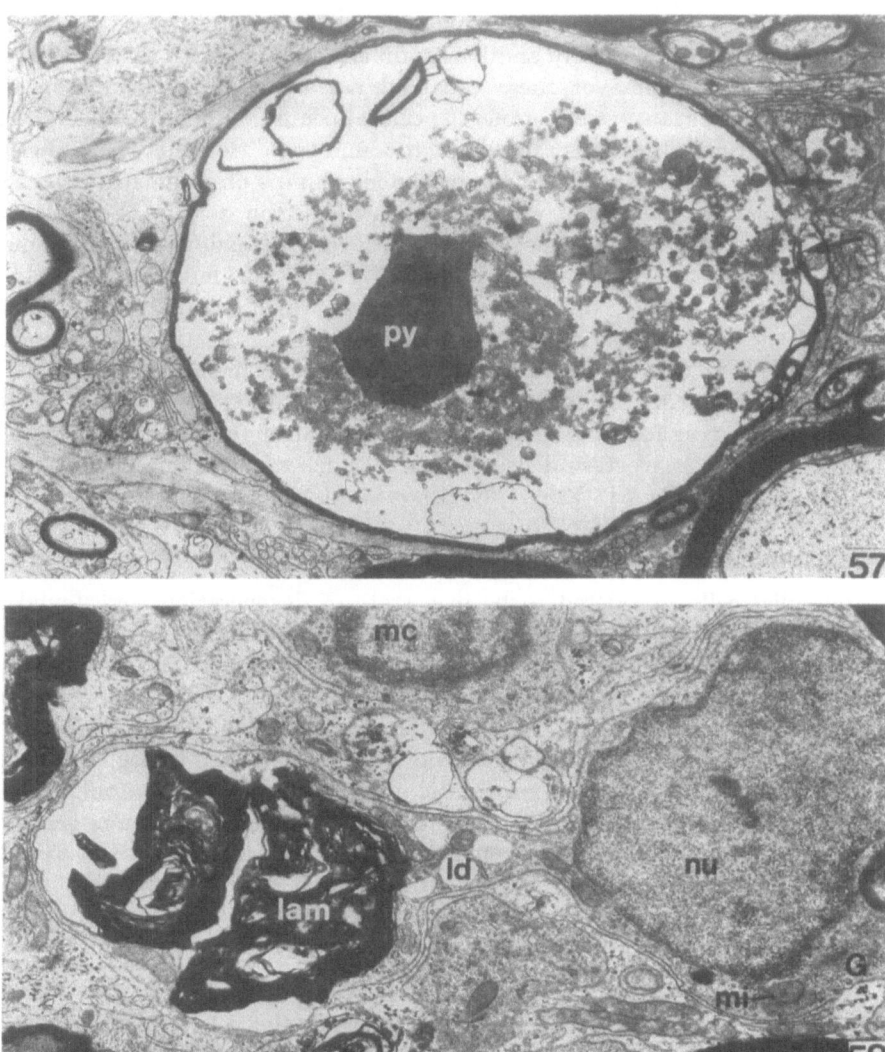

Fig. 56. 11 days at operation, 3 days survival. Longitudinal section. Degenerating glial cell. Structure interpreted as remnants of the nucleus shows a partially electron-dense and partially granular appearance. The presumed nuclear membrane (arrow) is largely intact. What is probably remnants of the cytoplasm show a granular appearance and contain a few dense bodies (*db*). A thin and irregular, but complete covering of myelin (*my*) is seen around the cell remnants. × 14200

Fig. 57. 17 days at operation, 23 days survival. Remnants of degenerating glial cell. The pyknotic nucleus can be seen (*py*). The membranous systems in the cytoplasm are severely deranged. The thin myelin which covers the cell remnants is incomplete, due to disruption of the myelin lamellae (arrows). × 8000

Fig. 58. 7 days at operation, 7 days survival. Longitudinal section. Microglial cell with a moderately electron-dense nucleus (*nu*), which is slightly irregular. The cytoplasm is less electron-dense than the nucleus and contains lamellar formations (*lam*), probably representing degenerating myelin, lipid droplets (*ld*), mitochondria with distinct cristae and Golgi apparatus (*G*). Above part of the nucleus and cytoplasm of another microglial cell (*mc*). × 9800 cells were most frequently seen at the 2-day stage. They were covered by myelin both in sections cut transversely and longitudinally in relation to the root fibres. Serial sections from some of these cells did not reveal any opening in the myelin covering. In transverse sections the cells appeared round or oval (Figs. 53, 55) and in longitudinal sections the cells were found to be elongated. The nucleus had an irregular outline and usually conspicuous clumps of chromatin (Fig. 53). The often abundant cytoplasm was of moderate electron density (Figs. 53, 55) and contained scattered ribosomes, a poorly developed endoplasmic reticulum (Figs. 53, 55), lipid droplets, dense bodies (Fig. 55), few mitochondria which often had distinct cristae, and a Golgi apparatus which was occasionally conspicuous. From the cytoplasm processes emerged which sometimes invaginated the parent cell (Fig. 53). Intracellular double or single unit membranes were sometimes observed (Fig. 55). Membrane-bounded bodies, often of a very irregular outline (Fig. 54) were found in some of these cells. Most frequently the content of these bodies was an electron-dense matrix in which rounded mitochondria-like structures occurred (Fig. 54). Rarely, bodies with a lamellated content or containing granular and vesiculated profiles could be seen. Structures resembling autophagosomes were not observed with certainty.

A few glial cells considered to be in a state of degeneration were found in most cases with survival times from 2 to 23 days. In two animals with survival times within this range such cells were not observed. At the 2-day stage degenerating glial cells were rarely found, while from 3 to 10 days they were more numerous. In no case, however, were they as numerous as in many cases of the previous study on indirect Wallerian degeneration of the kitten hypoglossal nerve (see Part I). A totally or partially pyknotic nucleus was consistenly found in the degenerating glial cells (Figs. 56, 57). In the greatly deranged cytoplasm granular profiles (Fig. 56) and membranous remnants (Fig. 57) were common features. As a rule these cells were covered by myelin and serial sections through some of these cells did not show any opening in this covering myelin. Around glial cells, which were obviously at an advanced stage of degeneration, the covering myelin was incomplete (Fig. 57).

Inclusion-containing cells without any myelin covering and resembling microglial cells described in the intramedullary root fibre region of the normal kitten hypoglossal nerve (see Part I) were seen in increased numbers from 6 days after operation. From 7 to 10 days they were a prominent feature of the process of degeneration. The nucleus of these cells was irregular with often peripherally located clumps of chromatin (Fig. 58). The cytoplasm was often scanty and less electron-dense than the nucleus (Fig. 58). A moderate number of free ribosomes, a few stacks of endoplasmic reticulum, mitochondria with distinct cristae, lipid inclusions (sometimes numerous) and phagocytosed fragments of degenerating myelinated nerve fibres were typical for these cells (Fig. 58). The phagocytosed structure usually consisted of myelin sheath fragments (Fig. 58), but myelinated electron-dense axoplasmic fragments were occasionally observed. No pictures indicating phagocytosis of degenerating glial cells were seen.

10 days after the operation there seemed to be an increase in the number of filament-filled astrocytic processes and by 23 days this increase was quite evident

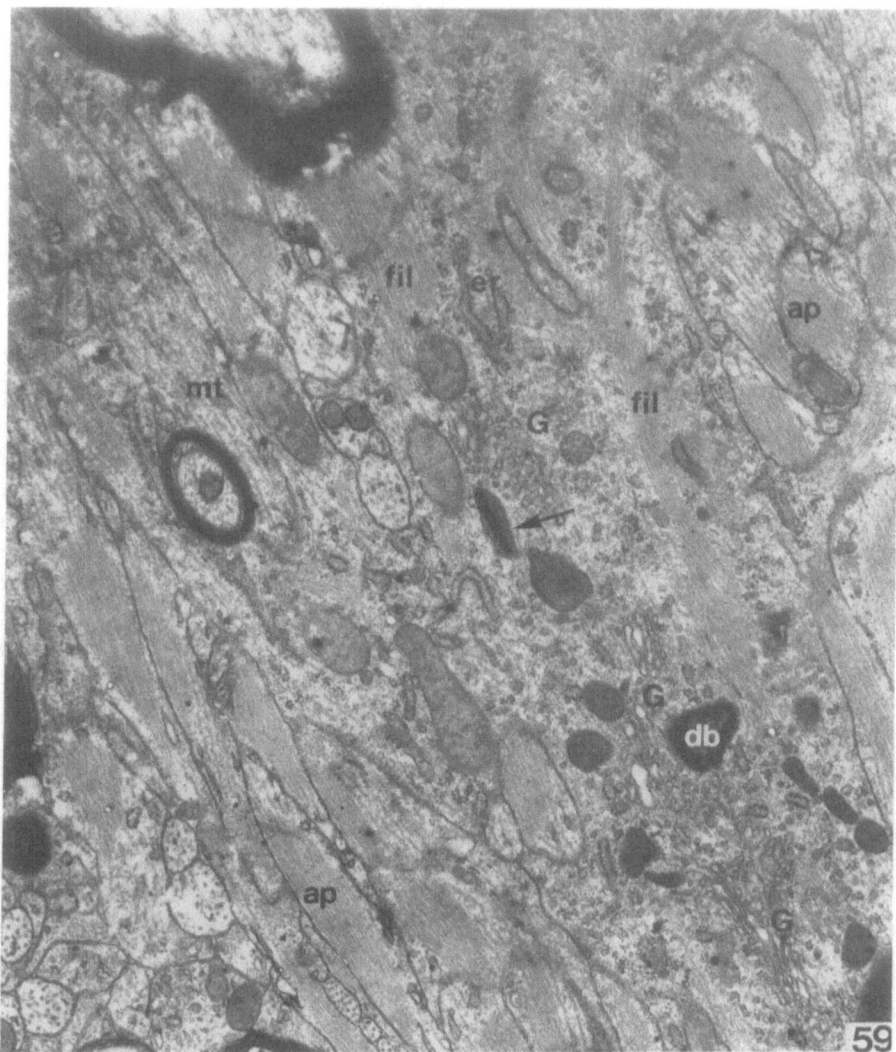

Fig. 59. 17 days at operation, 23 days survival. Longitudinal section. Part of hypertrophic astrocyte. The cytoplasm has numerous filaments (*fil*), a few microtubules (*mt*), a prominent Golgi apparatus (*G*), several dense bodies (*db*), one of which has a heterogenous appearance (arrow). Groups of ribosomes are rather densely packed between other cell organelles. The rough-surfaced endoplasmic reticulum (*er*) consists of a few scattered rows of membranes. The glial cell is surrounded by numerous astrocytic processes (*ap*) filled with filaments and a few microtubules. × 12000

in some parts of the intramedullary root fibre region (Fig. 58). At that stage the cytoplasm of many astrocytes was abundant and contained an unusual number of cell organelles, e.g. ribosomes, endoplasmic reticulum, Golgi apparatus and dense bodies (Fig. 59). Gliosomes of moderate size were frequently observed (Fig. 59). The astrocytic reaction was not as prominent as that during indirect

Wallerian degeneration in the intramedullary root fibre region of the hypoglossal nerve (see Part I). It should be noted, however, that in the present study
the animal with the longest survival time had only a small lesion of the hypoglossal nucleus (cf. Table 3).

Pericytes with a great number of vacuoles and dense bodies were observed
around some vessels adjacent to the intramedullary root fibres of the hypoglossal
nerve from 6 to 10 days. Similar cells were also observed around vessels lying
several 100 microns from these fibres.

IV. Discussion

Limitations Inherent in the Methods

Preparatory artifacts and "spontaneous" degeneration are two factors which
might have caused or contributed to the type of postoperative changes described
here. These factors were discussed in a previous study (see Part I). It was
concluded that preparatory artifacts were unlikely as a cause of the principal
changes observed in that study and that "spontaneous" degeneration could constitute only a small part of the degenerative changes on the operated side. These
conclusions are considered to be valid for the present investigation, too. Some
additional circumstances which have to be borne in mind when interpreting the
results of the present experiments are the short distance between the lesion and
the region studied, the differing extent of the lesions and the possible effect on
the degenerative process of postoperative edema, cerebrospinal fluid (CSF) leakage
or interference with the vascular supply.

Close to the site of lesion of a nerve fibre changes constituting a traumatic
reaction occurs which are not included in the term Wallerian degeneration. These
changes seem to extend 1–2 mm from the site of lesion (Cajal, 1928b; Zelená, 1969;
Schlote, 1970). To avoid studying traumatic changes care was taken in excluding
the area close to the lesion. No changes were observed corresponding to those
previously described as characteristic of the traumatic reaction (see e.g. Schlote).
Furthermore, the changes described here were observed in sections from proximal
as well as distal root fibre regions. Thus, it seems justifiable to conclude that the
principal changes described here are to be ascribed to a Wallerian type of
degeneration.

Since it was not possible to make the lesions in different animals identical
in terms of extent and localization (cf. Table 3), the number and distribution of
intramedullary root fibres affected inevitably differed in the various animals.
Moreover, since many cell bodies were probably affected some time after the
operation, due to bleeding and/or edema, the actual time of the interruption
in continuity between soma and axon is not known. The limitations imposed
by these factors with regard to exact timing and semiquantitative aspects, must
be borne in mind when interpreting the results of this study.

Postoperative edema and alterations in the CSF pressure might influence
the appearance of the degenerative changes. No changes indicative of edema in
the central nervous system (see e.g. Hirano, 1969) were found, however. Nor were
changes characteristic for the demyelinating lesions associated with CSF lesions
in the cat spinal cord (Bunge *et al.*, 1960) observed. Direct interference with the

vascular supply of the intramedullary root fibre region seems unlikely, since the vessels supplying this region come from the ventral side of the medulla. It is concluded that the factors discussed here are unlikely as causes of the *principal* changes observed in the present study. However, a negative effect by these factors on the penetration of the fixative solution cannot be excluded. It is possible that the difficulties in achieving an altogether satisfactory preservation can largely be attributed to these factors.

The advantages of the present study is that it has been performed on the same fibre system and animals of the same age range as was the previous study on indirect Wallerian degeneration (see Part I). This makes it possible to compare the principal features in this and the previous study without having to consider regional or maturational differences.

Comparison Between Morphological Changes during Direct and Indirect Wallerian Degeneration

At 6 and 20 hours after operation a few axons were seen with centrally placed tightly packed filaments and peripheral mitochondria, vesicles and lamellated profiles (Fig. 48). These axonal changes were not seen during indirect Wallerian degeneration (see Part I). They resemble some previously described early axonal changes in association with direct Wallerian degeneration in adult rats (Nathaniel and Nathaniel, 1973). However, the changes observed here to some extent also resemble previously described changes in the border zone of a nerve fibre where the traumatic reaction ends and the Wallerian degeneration starts (see e.g. Zelená, 1969). The axonal changes observed here may represent an unusually distant extension of the traumatic reaction in some nerve fibres. Alternatively, the changes could constitute an early stage in the process of direct Wallerian degeneration. The nerve fibres with tightly packed filaments and tubules, which were seen 20 hours postoperatively (Fig. 49) resemble some early axonal changes described in the previous study on indirect Wallerian degeneration (see Part I).

Electron-dense axons constituted the most conspicuous feature of axonal degeneration. Such axons have been reported during direct Wallerian degeneration in the retino-geniculate system of the kitten (Pecci Saavedra *et al.*, 1973) and in the kitten spinal cord (Hildebrand, 1971 b) and are also a well known feature of direct Wallerian degeneration in adult animals (see e.g. Lampert, 1967; McMahan, 1967; Mugnaini *et al.*, 1967; Dunkerley and Duncan, 1969). The morphology of the electron-dense axons observed in the present study corresponded well with such axons described during indirect Wallrian degeneration (see Part I).

Myelin bodies and aberrant myelin of a similar type as observed in the present study were noticed in the kitten spinal cord after dorsal root transections (Hildebrand, 1971 b). Similar changes have been observed in association with direct Wallerian degeneration in adult animals (see e.g. Lampert and Cressman, 1966; McMahan, 1967; Mugnaini *et al.*, 1967; Bignami and Ralston, 1969). The myelin sheath changes described in the previous study on indirect Wallerian degeneration coincide with those observed here. Thus, it is concluded that the

5*

principal degenerative changes in myelinated nerve fibres are the same in direct
and indirect Wallerian degeneration.

At the time when electron-dense axons became numerous, glial cells were found
which resembled microglial cells but were completely covered by myelin
(Figs. 53, 55). The general morphology of the cells, their complete envelopment
by myelin and their appearance early during the degenerative process all coincide
with previous observations made on myelin-covered microglial cells during indirect
Wallerian degeneration (see Part I). The latter seemed to have as a function
the phagocytosis of degenerating axoplasm. The present finding of membrane-
bounded bodies resembling degenerating axoplasm in the cytoplasm of some of
the microglial cells covered by myelin (Fig. 54), indicates a similar function for
these cells. At least some of these glial cells probably degenerate, since degenerating glial cells completely or partially covered by myelin (Figs. 11 and 12)
appeared at a time when myelin-covered microglial cells became infrequent
(cf. Diagram 2). Again, similar findings have been made during indirect Wallerian
degeneration (see Part I). Thus, on the basis of similarities of internal structure,
position and temporal relation to the degenerative process, as well as possible
similarities in function and fate, it is inferred that the myelin-covered microglial
cells described in this and in the previous study belong to the same category
of cell.

It seems likely that the microglial cells covered by myelin briefly mentioned
by Hildebrand (1971 b) in connection with direct Wallerian degeneration in the
kitten spinal cord, are identical to those described here. Probably, the same holds
true for the degenerating glial cells noticed in the study of Hildebrand (1971 b).
For both the myelin-covered microglial cells and the degenerating glial cells
observed here, the present study seems to be the first, however, to provide information concerning their detailed morphology, the time course of their occurrence,
their complete envelopment by myelin as well as their possible functional significance and fate.

The present findings rule out the possibility that indirect Wallerian degeneration might differ basically from direct Wallerian degeneration in the kitten with
regard to the myelin-covered microglial cells. It still remains an open question,
however, whether such cells as well as degenerating glial cells of the type
described here, are also an important feature of direct Wallerian degeneration
in adult cats. In the previous paper some earlier studies on direct Wallerian
degeneration in adult animals were discussed in which glial cells covered by
myelin and degenerating glial cells had been observed (see Part I). It was
noted that although some light microscopical studies on that process had yielded
findings which appeared to correlate rather well with the ultrastructural findings
on myelin-covered microglial cells and degenerating glial cells during indirect
Wallerian degeneration, electron microscopical studies have not convincingly
demonstrated the occurrence of similar types of cells during direct Wallerian
degeneration in adult animals. The present findings seem to call for a re-examina-
tion of the early glial reaction during direct Wallerian degeneration in such
animals.

Although no major qualitative differences were detected with regard to
myelin-covered microglial cells and degenerating glial cells between direct and

indirect Wallerian degeneration, the possibility of quantitative differences must be considered and in point of fact receives some support from the present study. Thus, myelin-covered microglial cells were common only in animals having survived for 2 days under the present experimental conditions—a very short period of time when comparing the situation in indirect Wallerian degeneration, where such cells were common from 5 to 15 days postoperatively (see Part I). It is also noteworthy that in contrast to what was found in the previous study on indirect Wallerian degeneration autophagosome-like structures were not observed with certainty in myelin-covered microglial cells in the present study. Moreover, degenerating glial cells were not as frequently seen in the present study as in the previous study on indirect Wallerian degeneration. It is not possible to say whether these observations reflect true differences between the two processes of Wallerian degeneration or are due to sources or error in the methods employed (see above).

Cells resembling the microglial cells seen in the normal intramedullary root fibre region of the hypoglossal nerve and located outside myelin were found to phagocytose fragments of degenerating myelinated nerve fibres. These phago-cytic cells appeared at a later stage than the myelin-covered microglial cells (cf. Diagram 2). Both these findings correspond to previous observations on indirect Wallerian degeneration in the kitten (see Part I). Also, the phagocytosing micro-glial cells located outside myelin seen in the present kitten material have a similar appearance as phagocytic cells described in some previous studies on direct Wallerian degeneration in adult animals (see e.g. Bignami and Ralston, 1969; Vaughn et al., 1970).

Corresponding observations were made in this and the preceding study (see Part I) with regard to the astrocytic reaction. In both instances hypertrophic astrocytes containing increased numbers of many cell organelles appeared in parallel with a proliferation of astrocytic processes. Probably as a result of the small size of the lesion of the hypoglossal nucleus in the "long-term" animal in the present study, this reaction was not as prominent as that observed during indirect Wallerian degeneration.

Pericytes seemed to be reactive in the present situation not only when situated adjacent to the intramedullary root fibres, but also far from them. It seems difficult to ascribe this reaction to the process of Wallerian degeneration in the intramedullary root fibres alone. The possibility of a generalized reaction of pericytes with the experimental procedure used here should be considered, in view of the generalized reaction of such cells described in some other situations, e.g. in association with a local freeze-injury of the brain (Cancilla et al., 1972) and after systemic injection of protein (Kristensson and Olsson, 1973).

The Rate of Wallerian Degeneration

The first signs of degeneration in the intramedullary root fibres of the kitten hypoglossal nerve were observed earlier in direct than in indirect Wallerian degeneration (see Part I). Since indirect Wallerian degeneration is preceded by a retrograde degeneration of the parent cell body (cf. van Gehuchten, 1903; Grant and Aldskogius, 1967) this finding could be anticipated. Compared to direct Wallerian degeneration the time course of indirect Wallerian degeneration in the root fibres is certainly more extended. Thus, electron-dense axons appeared 20 hours after the operation in the present study and were numerous 2 days postoperatively, while such axons in even younger animals appeared at 3 days but occurred with greatest frequency 9 to 15 days postoperatively (see Part I). Moreover, phagocytosis of myelin started 6 days after the operation in the present study and was prominent 7 days postoperatively, while during indirect Wallerian degeneration corresponding findings were made 9 days and 2 to 3 weeks after the operation respectively (see Part I). One reason for this difference is most likely that during the latter process the parent cells giving rise to the degenerating nerve fibres degenerate during a much longer time period than during the first process. Another reason may be that indirect and direct Wallerian degeneration in a given nerve fibre proceeds at different rates, being relatively slower during indirect Wallerian degeneration.

Electron microscopical studies on direct Wallerian degeneration of retino-geniculate fibres indicate that the rate of axonal degeneration is more rapid in kittens than in adult cats (Pecci Saavedra et al., 1973). In earlier light micro-scopical studies on direct Wallerian degeneration in the rabbit spinal cord, it was shown than the whole process of Wallerian degeneration runs a more rapid course in immature than in mature animals (Spatz, 1921). The present study seems to support both these observations. The findings of electron-dense axons 20 hours postoperatively, phagocytosis of myelin 6 days and a scar-forming astrocytic reaction 23 days postoperatively were all made significantly earlier than equi-valent previous findings in direct Wallerian degeneration of adult animals (see e.g. Bignami and Ralston, 1969; Dunkerly and Duncan, 1969; Vaughn et al., 1970; Vaughn and Pease, 1970). Results obtained in the course of previous electron microscopical studies on direct Wallerian degeneration in adult animals are not directly comparable to the present results, however, because of differences in the distance left between the site of lesion and the area studied, differences in the type of lesion and possible regional differences.

Concluding Remarks

The present study has shown that the principal changes distal as well as proximal to the site of nerve fibre lesion are qualitatively the same. This further supports previous suggestions to include the degenerative changes proximal to the site of nerve fibre lesion in the term Wallerian degeneration (van Gehuchten, 1903; Grant and Aldskogius, 1967; Grant, 1970).

While the present study has emphasized the morphological similarities between direct and indirect Wallerian degeneration in the kitten, it might in future studies be worthwhile exploring the possible quantitative differences between these two processes (see above). Assuming the existence of such differences, they are probably to a large extent attributable to the different relationship between parent cell body and degenerating nerve fibre in the two situations. While the distal portion of the nerve fibre (i.e. the one undergoing direct Wallerian degeneration) is more or less instantaneously disconnected from the parent cell body, the proximal part of the nerve fibre (i.e. the one undergoing indirect Wallerian degeneration) is most likely continuous with the parent cell body for some time after the nerve fibre lesion, thus allowing the parent cell body to exert important influences on the nerve fibre until this continuity is broken. It would be of particular interest if experiments could be deviced to test whether the rate of degeneration in a given nerve fibre is slower during indirect Wallerian degeneration compared to direct Wallerian degeneration. The existence of such a difference might render indirect Wallerian degeneration a suitable model for studying the process of Wallerian degeneration *per se*, since the extended time course would facilitate study of relatively short-lived changes.

V. Summary

The ultrastructural changes occurring distal to a nerve fibre lesion, so-called direct Wallerian degeneration, have been studied in the intramedullary root fibre region of the kitten hypoglossal nerve 6 hours to 23 days after unilateral lesions of the hypoglossal nucleus.

6 to 20 hours after the operation axons are found with tightly packed filaments located centrally and vesicles, mitochondria and lamellar formations peripherally. Electron-dense axons (a sign of axonal degeneration) are occasionally observed 20 hours postoperatively and frequently observed 2 to 10 days postoperatively. Signs of myelin sheath degeneration, mainly in the form of myelin bodies occur from 2 to 23 days.

At an early stage of the degenerative process microglial cells completely covered by myelin are found. These cells seem to participate in the pagocytosis of degenerating axoplasm. At a somewhat later stage degenerating glial cells completely or partially covered by myelin appear. Fragments of degenerating myelinated nerve fibres are phagocytosed by microglial cells located outside myelin. Concomitant with the disappearance of the degenerating nerve fibres, hypertrophic astrocytes and increased numbers of astrocytic processes are observed.

The results are discussed in relation to previous findings on indirect Wallerian degeneration in the same nerve fibre system of the kitten. It is concluded that the principal ultrastructural changes are the same in direct as in indirect Wallerian degeneration in this system of the kitten. Of particular relevance is that a certain type of myelin-covered microglial cells, prominent during indirect Wallerian degeneration, have for the first time been implicated in the process of direct Wallerian degeneration.

Acknowledgement. My sincere thanks are due to Professor G. Grant, M. D. Department of Anatomy, Karolinska Institutet, Stockholm, for his constant encouragement and support during the course of this study.

The constructive criticism of the manuscript by Drs. C. Hildebrand and Renée Schild is gratefully acknowledged.

Excellent technical assistance was given by Miss Maj Berghman, Mrs. Siv Blomquist, Mrs. Gunvor Pettersson and Miss Brita Robertsson.

This work was supported by grants from the Swedish Medical Research Council (Project nos. B71-12X-553-07C, B72-12X-553-08A and B73-12X-553-09B) and from Karolinska Instituted.

References

Aguayo, A. J., Terry, L. C., Bray, G. M.: Spontaneous loss of axons in sympathetic unmyelinated nerve fibres of the rat during development. Brain Res. **54**, 360–364 (1973)

Aldskogius, H.: Indirect Wallerian fiber degeneration in the hypoglossal nerve of the kitten. An electron microscopical study. J. Ultrastruct. Res. **42**, 409 (1973)

Arstila, A. U., Trump, B. F.: Studies on cellular autophagocytosis. The formation of auto-phagic vacuoles in the liver after glucagon administration. Amer. J. Path. **53**, 687–733 (1968)

Barron, K. D., Doolin, P. F.: Ultrastructural observations on retrograde atrophy of lateral geniculate body. II. The environs of the neuronal soma. J. Neuropath. exp. Neurol. **27**, 401–420 (1968)

Barron, K. D., Means, E. D., Larsen, E.: Ultrastructure of retrograde degeneration in thalamus of rat. I. Neuronal somata and dendrites. J. Neuropath. exp. Neurol. **32**, 218–244 (1973)

Beresford, W. A.: A discussion on retrograde changes in nerve fibres. pp. 33–56. In: Progr. in Brain Res. Vol. 14. Degeneration patterns in the nervous system. Eds. M. Singer and J. P. Schadé. Amsterdam: Elsevier 1965

Berger, B.: Etude ultrastructurale de la dégénéresence wallérienne expérimentale d'un nerf entièrement amyélinique: le nerf olfactif. II. Réactions cellulaires. J. Ultrastruct. Res. **37**, 479–494 (1971)

Berthold, C.-H.: A study on the fixation of large mature feline myelinated ventral lumbar spinal-root fibres. Acta Soc. Med. upsalien. **73**, suppl. 9 (1968)

Berthold, C.-H., Skoglund, S.: Postnatal development of feline paranodal myelin-sheath segments. I. Light microscopy. Acta Soc. Med. upsalien. **73**, 113–126 (1968a)

Berthold, C.-H., Skoglund, S.: Postnatal development of feline paranodal myelin-sheath segments. II. Electron microscopy. Acta Soc. Med. upsalien. **73**, 127–144 (1968b)

Bignami, A., Ralston, H. J. III: Myelination of fibrillary astroglial processes in long term Wallerian degeneration. The possible relationship to status marmoratus. Brain Res. **11**, 710–713 (1968)

Bignami, A., Ralston, H. J. III.: The cellular reaction to Wallerian degeneration in the central nervous system of the cat. Brain Res. **13**, 444–461 (1969)

Blakemore, W. F.: The ultrastructure of the subependymal plate in the rat. J. Anat. (Lond.) **104**, 423–433 (1969)

Blakemore, W. F.: Microglial reactions following thermal necrosis of the rat cortex: An electron microscope study. Acta neuropath. (Berl.) **21**, 11–22 (1972a)

Blakemore, W. F.: Observations on oligodendrocyte degeneration, the resolution of status spongiosus and remyelination in cuprizone intoxication in mice. J. Neurocytol. **1**, 413–426 (1972b)

Blakemore, W. F., Palmer, A. C., Noel, P. R. B.: Ultrastructural changes in isoniazid-induced brain oedema in the dog. J. Neurocytol. **1**, 263–278 (1972)

Bodian, D.: Spontaneous degeneration in the spinal cord of monkey fetuses. Bull. Johns Hopk. Hosp. **119**, 212–234 (1966)

Bregman, E.: Über experimentelle aufsteigende Degeneration motorischer und sensibler Hirnnerven. Arb. neurol. Inst. Univ. Wien **1**, 73–97 (1892)

Brodal, A.: Experimentelle Untersuchungen über retrograde Zellveränderungen in der unteren Olive nach Läsionen des Kleinhirns. Z. ges. Neurol. Psychiat. **166**, 646–704 (1939)

Brownson, R. H., Ingersoll, E. H., Carsten, A. L.: Fine-structure of bilateral radionecrosis in the dorsal hippocampus. Acta neuropath. (Berl.) **21**, 89–98 (1972)

Bunge, R. P.: Glial cells and the central myelin sheath. Physiol. Rev. **48**, 197–251 (1968)

Bunge, R. P., Bunge, M. B., Ris, H.: Electron microscopic study of demyelination in an experimentally induced lesion in adult cat spinal cord. J. biophys. biochem. Cytol. **7**, 685–696 (1960)

Cajal, S. R. y: Degeneration and regeneration of the nervous system. Vol. I. New York: Hafner Publ. Co. 1928a

Cajal, S. R. y: Degeneration and regeneration of the nervous system. Vol. II. New York: Hafner Publ. Co. 1928b

Cancilla, P. A., Baker, R. N., Pollock, P. S., Frommes, S. P.: The reaction of pericytes of the central nervous system to exogenous protein. Lab. Invest. **26**, 376–383 (1972)

Cavanagh, J. B.: The proliferation of astrocytes around a needle wound in the rat brain. J. Anat. (Lond.) **106**, 471–487 (1970)

Cole, M.: Retrograde degeneration of axon and soma in the nervous system. pp. 269–300. In: Structure and Function of Nervous Tissue Ed. G. H. Bourne Vol. I. New York, London: Acad. Press. 1968

Cole, M., Nauta, W. J. H.: Retrograde atrophy of axons of the medial lemniscus of the cat. An experimental study. J. Neuropath. exp. Neurol. **29**, 354–369 (1970)

Cowan, W. M., Adamson, L., Powell, T. P. S.: An experimental study of the avian visual system. J. Anat. (Lond.) **95**, 545–563 (1961)

Cramer, F., Alpers, B. J.: The functions of the glia in secondary degeneration of the spinal cord. Arch Pathol. **13**, 23–55 (1932)

Cupédo, R. N. J.: Indirect Wallerian degeneration of afferents from the masticatory muscles. Acta morph. neerl.-scand. **8**, 101–118 (1970)

Cravioto, H.: Wallerian degeneration: ultrastructural and histochemical studies. Bull. Los Angeles neurol. Soc. **34**, 233–253 (1969)

Dalton, M. M., Hommes, O. R., Leblond, C. P.: Correlation of glial proliferation with age in the mouse brain. J. comp. Neurol. **134**, 397–400 (1968)

Daniel, P. M., Strich, S. J.: Histological observations on Wallerian degeneration in the spinal cord of the baboon, Papio papio. Acta neuropath. (Berl.) **12**, 314–328 (1969)

Das, G. D., Hine, R. J.: Nature and significance of spontaneous degeneration of axons in the pyramidal tract. Z. Anat. Entwickl.-Gesch. **136**, 98–114 (1972)

De Duve, C., Wattiaux, R.: Functions of lysosomes. Ann. Rev. Physiol. **28**, 435–492 (1966)

Dunkerley, G. B., Duncan, D.: A light and electron microscopic study of the normal and degenerating corticospinal tract in the rat. J. comp. Neurol. **137**, 155–184 (1969)

Eager, R. P., Barrnett, R. J.: Morphological and chemical studies of Nauta-stained degenerating cerebellar and hypothalamic fibers. J. comp. Neurol. **126**, 487–510 (1966)

Ericsson, J. L. E.: Mechanism of cellular autophagy. pp. 345–394. In: Lysosomes in biology and pathology. Vol. 2. Eds. J. T. Dingle and H. B. Fell. Amsterdam North-Holland Publ. Co. 1969

Ericsson, J. L. E., Trump, B. F., Weibel, J.: Electron microscopic studies of proximal tubule of the rat kidney. II. Cytosegrosomes and cytosomes. Their relationship to each other and to the lysosome concept. Lab. Invest. **14**, 1341–1365 (1965)

Fedorko, M. E., Hirsch, J. G., Cohn, Z. A.: Autophagic vacuoles produced in vitro. II. Studies on the mechanism of formation of autophagic vacuoles produced by chloroquine. J. Cell Biol. **38**, 392–402 (1968)

Fleischauer, K., Schmalbach, K.: Vergleichende Untersuchungen über die Reaktionsweise des jugendlichen und des erwachsenen Gehirnes nach intracerebraler Injektion von Aluminiumhydroxyd. Acta neuropath. (Berl.) **11**, 311–329 (1968)

Fox, H.: Degeneration of the nerve cord in the tail of Rana temporaria during metamorphic climax: study by electron microscopy. J. Embryol. exp. Morph. **30**, 377–396 (1973)

Friede, R. L.: Enzyme histochemistry of neuroglia. pp. 35–47. In: Progr. in Brain Res. Vol. 15. Biology of Neuroglia. Eds. E. D. P. de Robertis and R. Carrea. Amsterdam: Elsevier 1965

Gehuchten, A. van: La dégénérescence dite rétrograde ou dégénérescence Wallérienne indirecte. Névraxe **5**, 3–107 (1903)

Glees, P., Soler, J., Bailey, R. A.: Retrograde axonal changes of the deafferentated nucleus gracilis following mid-brain tractotomy. J. Neurol. Neurosurg. Psychiat. **14**, 281–286 (1951)

Glinsmann, W. H., Ericsson, J. L. E.: Observations on the subcellular organization of hepatic parenchymal cells. II. Evolution of reversible alterations induced by hypoxia. Lab. Invest. **15**, 762–777 (1966)

Grant, G.: Silver impregnation of degenerating dendrites, cells and axons central to axonal transection. II. A Nauta study on spinal motor neurones in kittens. Exp. Brain Res. **6**, 284–293 (1968)

Grant, G.: Neuronal changes central to the site of axon transection. A method for the identification of retrograde changes in perikarya, dendrites and axons by silver impregnation. pp. 173–185. In: Contemporary Research Methods in Neuroanatomy. Eds. W. J. H. Nauta and S. O. E. Ebbeson. Berlin, Heidelberg, New York: Springer 1970

Grant, G., Aldskogius, H.: Silver impregnation of degenerating dendrites, cells and axons central to axonal transection. I. A Nauta study on the hypoglossal nerve in kittens. Exp. Brain Res. **3**, 150–162 (1967)

Grant, G., Westman, J.: The lateral cervical nucleus in the cat. IV. A light and electron microscopical study after midbrain lesions with demonstration of indirect Wallerian degeneration at the ultra-structural level. Exp. Brain Res. **7**, 51–67 (1969)

Gray, E. G., Hamlyn, L. H.: Electron microscopy of experimental degeneration in the avian optic tectum. J. Anat. (Lond.) **96**, 309–316 (1962)

Guillery, R. W.: Patterns of fiber degeneration in the dorsal lateral geniculate nucleus of the cat following lesions in the visual cortex. J. comp. Neurol. **130**, 197–222 (1967)

Guillery, R. W.: Light—and electron—microscopical studies of normal and degenerating axons. pp. 77–105. In: Contemporary Research methods in Neuroanatomy. Eds. W. J. H. Nauta and S. O. E. Ebbeson. Berlin-Heidelberg-New York: Springer 1970

Guth, L., Watson, P. K.: A correlated histochemical and quantitative study on cerebral glycogen after brain injury in the rat. Exp. Neurol. **22**, 590–602 (1968)

Hayat, M. A.: Principles and techniques of electron microscopy. Biological applications. Vol. 1. New York: Van Nostrand Reinhold Co. 1970

Heimer, L., Ekholm, R.: Neuronal argyrophilia in early degenerative states: a light and electron microscopic study of the Glees and Nauta techniques. Experientia **23**, 237–239 (1967)

Heimer, L., Peters, A.: An electron microscope study of a silver stain for degenerating boutons. Brain Res. **8**, 337–346 (1968)

Hildebrand, C.: Ultrastructural and light-microscopic studies of the nodal region in large myelinated fibres of the adult feline spinal cord white matter. Acta physiol. scand. suppl. **364**, 43–80 (1971 a)

Hildebrand, C.: Ultrastructural and light-microscopic studies of the developing feline spinal cord white matter. II. Cell death and myelin sheath disintegration in the early postnatal period. Acta physiol. scand. suppl. **364**, 109–144 (1971 b)

Hirano, A.: The fine structure of brain in edema. pp. 69–135. In: The Structure and Function of Nervous Tissue. Vol. II. Ed. G. H. Bourne. New York, London: Acad. Press. (1969)

Hommes, O. R., Leblond, C. P.: Mitotic division of neuroglia in the normal adult rat. J. comp. Neurol. **129**, 269–278 (1967)

Howell, J. I., Kidd, M.: An electron microscopical comparison of primary and secondary demyelination in the rat central nervous system. Virchows Arch., Abt. B **2**, 187–202 (1969)

Jakob, A.: Über die feinere Histologie der sekundären Faserdegeneration in der weißen Substanz des Rückenmarks (mit besonderer Berücksichtigung der Abbauvorgänge). Histol. Histopathol. Arb. Großhirnrinde **5**, 1–181 (1913)

Kitamura, T., Hattori, H., Fujita, S.: Autoradiographic studies on histogenesis of brain macrophages in the mouse. J. Neuropath. exp. Neurol. **31**, 502–518 (1972)

Konigsmark, B. W., Sidman, R. L.: Origin of brain macrophages in the mouse. J. Neuropath. exp. Neurol. **22**, 643–676 (1963)

Kristensson, K., Olsson, Y.: Accumulation of protein tracers in pericytes of the central nervous system following systemic injection in immature mice. Acta neurol. scand. **49**, 189–194 (1973)

Kruger, L., Maxwell, D. S.: Electron microscopy of oligodendrocytes in normal rat cerebrum. Amer. J. Anat. **118**, 411–436 (1966)

Lampert, P. W.: A comparative electron microscopic study of reactive degenerating, regenerating and dystrophic axons. J. Neuropath. exp. Neurol. **26**, 345–368 (1967 a)

Lampert, P. W.: Electron microscopic studies on ordinary and hyperacute experimental allergic encephalomyelitis. Acta neuropath. (Berl.) **9**, 99–126 (1967 b)

Lampert, P. W., Cressman, M. R.: Axonal regeneration in the dorsal columns of the spinal cord of adult rats. An electron microscopic study. Lab. Invest. **13**, 825–839 (1964)

Lampert, P. W., Cressman, M. R.: Fine-structural changes of myelin sheaths after axonal degeneration in the spinal cord of rats. Amer. J. Pathol. **49**, 1139–1155 (1966)

Lampert, P. W., Schochet, S. S.: Electron microscopic observations on experimental spongy degeneration of the cerebellar white matter. J. Neuropath. exp. Neurol. **27**, 210–220 (1968)

LaVelle, A., LaVelle, F. W.: The nucleolar apparatus and neuronal reactivity to injury during development. J. exp. Zool. **137**, 285–315 (1958)

Lodge, D., Duggan, A. W., Biscoe, T. J., Caddy, K. W. T.: Concerning recurrent collaterals and afferent fibres in the hypoglossal nerve of the rat. Exp. Neurol. **41**, 53–75 (1973)

Lyser, K. M.: The fine structure of glial cells in the chicken. J. comp. Neurol. **146**, 83–93 (1972)

Matthews, M. A., Kruger, L.: Electron microscopy of non-neuronal cellular changes accompanying neural degeneration in thalamic nuclei of the rabbit. II. Reactive elements within the neuropil. J. comp. Neurol. **148**, 313–346 (1973)

Maxwell, D. S., Kruger, L.: The fine structure of astrocytes in the cerebral cortex and their response to focal injury produced by heavy ionizing particles. J. Cell Biol. **25**, 141–157 (1965)

McMahan, U. J.: Fine structure of synapses in the dorsal nucleus of the lateral geniculate body of normal and blinded rats. Z. Zellforsch. **76**, 116–146 (1967)

Millonig, G.: Advantages of a phosphate buffer for OsO_4 solutions in fixation. J. appl. Physics. **32**, 1637 (1961)

Miquel, J., Haymaker, W.: Astroglial reaction to ionizing radiation with emphasis on glycogen accumulation. pp. 98–114. In: Progr. In Brain Res. Vol. 15. Eds. E. D. P., de Robertis and R. Carrea. Amsterdam: Elsevier 1965

Mori, S., Leblond, C. P.: Identification of microglia in light and electron microscopy. J. comp. Neurol. **135**, 57–79 (1969a)

Mori, S., Leblond, C. P.: Electron microscopic features and proliferation of astrocytes in the corpus callosum of the rat. J. comp. Neurol. **137**, 197–226 (1969b)

Mori, S., Leblond, C. P.: Electron microscopic identification of three classes of oligodendrocytes and a preliminary study of their proliferative activity in the corpus callosum of young rats. J. comp. Neurol. **139**, 1–30 (1970)

Morris, J. H., Hudson, A. R., Weddell, G.: A study of degeneration and regeneration in the divided rat sciatic nerve based on electron microscopy. III. Changes in the axons of the proximal stump. Z. Zellforsch. **124**, 131–164 (1972)

Mossakowski, M. J., Penar, B.: Some aspects of the histochemistry of the reactive glia. Neuropat. pol. **10**, 317–323 (1972)

Mugnaini, E.: The histology and cytology of the cerebellar cortex. pp. 201–264. In: The comparative anatomy and histology of the cerebellum. Eds. O. Larsell and J. Jansen. Minnesota: Univ. Minn. Press. 1972

Mugnaini, E., Walberg, F.: Ultrastructure of neuroglia. Ergebn. Anat. Entwickl.-Gesch. **37**, 194–236 (1964)

Mugnaini, E., Walberg, F.: An experimental electron microscopical study on the mode of termination of cerebellar corticovestibular fibres in the cat lateral vestibular nucleus (Deiter's nucleus). Exp. Brain Res. **4**, 212–236 (1967)

Mugnaini, E., Walberg, F., Brodal, A.: Mode of termination of primary vestibular fibres in the lateral vestibular nucleus. An experimental electron microscopical study in the cat. Exp. Brain Res. **4**, 187–211 (1967)

Muirhead, P. D., Mezei, C.: Pattern of RNA synthesis in the sciatic nerve of the hen during Wallerian degeneration. J. Neurochem. **21**, 147–158 (1973)

Nathaniel, E. J. H., Nathaniel, D. R.: Degeneration of dorsal roots in the adult rat spinal cord. Exp. Neurol. **40**, 316–332 (1973)

Nathaniel, E. J. H., Pease, D. C.: Degenerative changes in rat dorsal roots during Wallerian degeneration. J. Ultrastruct. Res. **9**, 511–532 (1963)

Oemichen, M., Grüninger, H., Saebisch, R., Narita, Y.: Mikroglia und Pericyten als Transformationsformen der Blut-Monocyten mit erhaltener Proliferationsfähigkeit. Experimentelle autoradiographische und enzymhistochemische Untersuchungen am normalen und geschädigten Kaninchen- und Rattengehirn. Acta neuropath. (Berl.) **23**, 200–218 (1973)

O'Neal, J. T., Westrum, L. E.: The fine structural synaptic organization of the cat lateral cuneate nucleus. A study of sequential alterations in degeneration. Brain Res. **51**, 97–124 (1973)

Pannese, E. Ferrannini, E.: Nuclear pyknosis in neuroglia cells of normal mammals. Acta neuropath. (Berl.) **8**, 309–319 (1967)

Pecci Saavedra, J., Mascitti, T. A., Pérez Lloret, I. L.: Increased rate of anterograde degeneration in the visual pathway of kittens. Brain Res. **50**, 265–274 (1973)

Peters, A., Palay, S. L., Webster, H. de F.: The fine structure of the nervous system. The cells and their processes. New York: Harper and Row Publ. 1970

Phillips, D. E.: An electron microscopic study of macroglia and microglia in the lateral funiculus of the developing spinal cord in the fetal monkey Z. Zellforsch. **140**, 145–167 (1973)

Powell, T. P. S., Cowan, W. M.: A note on retrograde fibre degeneration. J. Anat. (Lond.) **98**, 579–585 (1964)

Privat, A., Robain, O., Mandel, P.: Aspects ultrastructuraux du corps calleux chez la souris Jimpy. Acta neuropath. (Berl.) **21**, 282–295 (1972)

Raine, C. S., Bornstein, M. B.: Experimental allergic encephalitis: an ultrastructural study of experimental demyelination in vitro. J. Neuropath. exp. Neurol. **24**, 177–191 (1970)

Rand, C. W.: The role of the astrocyte in the formation of cerebral scars. Bull. Los Angeles neurol. Soc. **17**, 57–70 (1952)

Reier, P. J., Hughes, A.: Evidence for spontaneous axon degeneration during peripheral nerve maturation. Amer. J. Anat. **135**, 147–152 (1972)

Reynolds, E. S.: The use of lead citrate at high pH as an electron- opaque stain in electron microscopy. J. Cell Biol. **17**, 208–212 (1963)

Russel, G. V.: The compound granular corpuscle or gitter cell: a review, together with notes on the origin of this phagocyte. Tex. Rep. Biol. Med. **20**, 338–351 (1962)

Scharrer, B.: Ultrastructural study of the regressing prothoracic glands of Blattarian insects. Z. Zellforsch. **69**, 1–21 (1966)

Schlote, W.: Nervus opticus und experimentelles Trauma. Beitrag zur Cytologie und Cytopathologie eines zentralnervösen Markfasersystems. Monographien aus dem Gesamtgebiete der Neurologie und Psychiatrie. Heft 131. Berlin, Heidelberg, New York: Springer 1970

Shimizu, N., Hamuro, Y.: Deposition of glycogen and changes in some enzymes in brain wounds. Nature (Lond.) **181**, 609–611 (1958)

Skoff, R. P., Vaughn, J. E.: An autoradiographic study of cellular proliferation in degenerating rat optic nerve. J. comp. Neurol. **141**, 133–156 (1971)

Smart, I., Leblond, C. P.: Evidence for division and transformations of neuroglia cells in the mouse brain, as derived from radioautography after injection of Thymidine-H³. J. comp. Neurol. **116**, 349–367 (1961)

Spatz, H.: Beiträge zur normalen Histologie des Rückenmarks des neugeborenen Kaninchens mit Berücksichtigung der Veränderungen während der extrauterinen Entwicklung. Histol. Histopathol. Arb. Großhirnrinde **6**, 478–604 (1918)

Spatz, H.: Über die Vorgänge nach experimenteller Rückenmarksdurchtrennung mit besonderer Berücksichtigung der Unterschiede der Reaktionsweise des reifen und des unreifen Gewebes. pp. 49—364. In: Histol. Histopathol. Arb. Großhirnrinde. Jena: Gustav Fischer 1921

Stenwig, A. E.: The origin of brain macrophages in traumatic lesions, Wallerian degeneration, and retrograde degeneration. J. Neuropath. exp. Neurol. **31**, 696–704 (1972)

Sumi, S. M., Hager, H.: Electron microscopic study of the reaction of the newborn rat brain to injury. Acta neuropath. (Berl.) **10**, 324–335 (1968)

Suzuki, K., Andrews, J. M., Waltz, J. M., Terry, R. D.: Ultrastructural studies of Multiple Sclerosis. Lab. Invest. **20**, 444–454 (1969)

Suzuki, K.: La Dorna De Paul: Cellular degeneration in developing central nervous system of rats produced by hypocholesteremic drug AY 9944. Lab. Invest. **25**, 546–555 (1971)

Takano, I.: Electron microscopic studies on retrograde chromatolysis in the hypoglossal nucleus and changes in the hypoglossal nerve, following its severance and ligation. Okajimas Fol. anat. jap. **40**, 1–69 (1964)

Torvik, A.: Transneuronal changes in the inferior olive and pontine nuclei in kittens. J. Neuropath. exp. Neurol. **15**, 119–145 (1956)

Torvik, A., Skjörten, F.: Electron microscopic observations on nerve cell regeneration and degeneration after axon lesion. I. Changes in the nerve cell cytoplasm. Acta neuropath. (Berl.) **17**, 248–264 (1971)

Trump, B. F., Ericsson, J. L. E.: The effect of the fixative solution on the ultrastructure of cells and tissues. A comparative analysis with particular attention to the proximal convoluted tubule of the rat kidney. Lab. Invest. **14**, 1245–1323 (1965)

Trumpy, J. H.: Transneuronal degeneration in the pontine nuclei of the cat. Ergebn. Anat. Entwickl.-Gesch. **44**, 1–72 (1971)

Vaughn, J. E.: Electron microscopic study of the vascular response to axonal degeneration in rat optic nerve. Anat. Rec. **151**, 428 (1965)

Vaughn, J. E., Hinds, P. L., Skoff, R. P.: Electron microscopic studies of Wallerian degeneration in rat optic nerves. I. The multipotential glia. J. comp. Neurol. **140**, 175–206 (1970)

Vaughn, J. E., Pease, D. C.: Electron microscopic studies of Wallerian degeneration in rat optic nerves. II. Astrocytes, oligodendrocytes and adventitial cells. J. comp. Neurol. **140**, 207–226 (1970)

Vaughn, J. E., Peters, A.: A third neuroglial cell type. An electron microscopic study. J. comp. Neurol. **133**, 269–288 (1968)

Vaughn, J. E., Peters, A.: The morphology and development of neuroglial cells. pp. 103–140. In: Cellular aspects of neural growth and differentiation. Ed. D. C. Pease UCLA Forum Med. Sci. No. 14, Los Angeles: Univ. Calif. Press. 1971

Vaughn, J. E., Skoff, R. P.: Neuroglia in experimentally altered central nervous system. pp. 39–72. In: Structure and Function of Nervous Tissue. Vol. V. Ed. G. H. Bourne. New York, London: Acad Press. 1972

Walberg, F.: Does silver impregnate normal and degenerating boutons? A study based on light and electron microscopical observations of the inferior olive. Brain Res. **31**, 47–65 (1971)

Walberg, F.: Further studies on silver impregnation of normal and degenerating boutons. A light and electron microscopical investigation of a filamentous degenerating system. Brain Res. **36**, 353–369 (1972)

Wechsler, W., Hager, H.: Elektronenmikroskopische Untersuchungen der Wallerschen Degeneration des peripheren Säugetiernerven. Beitr. pathol. Anat. **126**, 352–380 (1962)

Wendell-Smith, C. P., Blund, M. J., Baldwin, F.: The ultrastructural characterization of macroglial cell types. J. comp. Neurol. **127**, 219–240 (1966)

Wong-Riley, M. T. T.: Changes in the dorsal lateral geniculate nucleus of the squirrel monkey after unilateral ablation of the visual cortex. J. comp. Neurol. **146**, 519–548 (1972)

Zelená, J.: Bidirectional shift of mitochondria in axons after injury. pp. 73–94. In: Cellular Dynamics of the Neuron. Ed. S. H. Barondes. New York-London: Acad. Press. 1969

Subject Index

Aberrant myelin, see Myelin
Astrocytes   15, 39, 48, 64, 69
Axonal degeneration, see Degeneration

Degeneration, axonal 16, 19, 42, 56, 67
—, glial cell   15, 17, 27, 45, 64, 68
—, myelin   15, 16, 21, 42, 56, 67
—, retrograde   7, 49, 50
—, "spontaneous"   41, 46
—, terminal   45
—, time course   69
—, transneuronal   46
—, traumatic   7, 48, 66
—, Wallerian, direct (definition)   8
—, —, indirect (definition)   7, 70
Demyelination   46
Development, postnatal   11, 41

Glial cell degeneration, see Degeneration
Gliosomes   39, 65
Glycogen   39, 48

Lamellated bodies (structures)   25, 31,
    43, 64
Lysosomes, autophagosomes   44
—, heterophagosomes   43, 44, 48

Membrane-bounded bodies (in myelin-
    covered microglial cells)   23, 43, 64, 68

Microglial cells, myelin-covered   21, 42,
    60, 68
—, outside myelin   15, 17, 21, 47, 64, 69
Mitosis (mitotic cells)   15, 21, 47
Myelin, aberrant   15, 21, 42, 60, 67
—, bodies   15, 21, 42, 56, 67
—, degeneration, see Degeneration
—, normal   11
Myeloclasts   44, 45, 46

Nauta method   7, 8, 50
Nodes of Ranvier   25, 42

Oligodendrocytes   11, 31, 41, 49

Pericytes   15, 31, 48, 66, 69
Preparation artifacts   39, 41, 67
Phagocytes, cell type   44, 47, 68, 69
—, origin   43, 47
Phagocytosis of, axoplasm   31, 43, 64, 68
—, glial cells   17, 31
—, myelin   15, 31, 43, 47, 64, 69
Pyknotic nucleus (body) see Degeneration,
    glial cell

Regeneration   49
Remyelination   49